Bearing Up
with cancer

Dr. Annie Smith

life and living with...

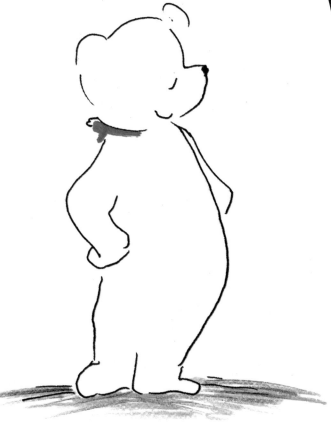

Second
Story
Press

NATIONAL LIBRARY OF CANADA
CATALOGUING IN PUBLICATION

Smith, Annie, 1940–
    Bearing up with cancer : life, and living with ... /
Annie Smith.

ISBN 1-896764-80-0

    1. Smith, Annie, 1940–   2. Cancer – Patients –
Biography. 3. Art teachers – Ontario – Mississauga –
Biography. 4. College teachers – Ontario – Mississauga –
Biography. I. Title.

RC265.6.S63A3 2004   362.1'96994'0092
C2003-905985-5

Edited by Susan Goldberg
Designed by Counterpunch / Linda Gustafson
Printed and bound in Canada

*Second Story Press gratefully acknowledges the support of the Ontario
Arts Council and the Canada Council for the Arts for our publishing
program. We acknowledge the financial support of the Government of
Canada through the Book Publishing Industry Development Program,
and the Government of Ontario through the Ontario Media
Development Corporation's Ontario Book Initiative.*

Published by
SECOND STORY PRESS
720 Bathurst Street, Suite 301
Toronto, Ontario, Canada
M5S 2R4

www.secondstorypress.on.ca

To my mom

Acknowledgments

I worried about writing a formal "acknowledg-
ment page." So many people have contributed
to my being here today that I feared I would
inadvertently leave someone out.

I wish to acknowledge those who have not lived
long enough to be part of my last twenty-plus
years, including my folks and my family, who have
so obviously contributed to my life.

I thank my wonderful friends and colleagues,
who have been so generous and supportive in
every way imaginable; my special surgeon /
gynecological oncologist and his medical team
and office assistants, who in their wisdom have
guided me through countless medical proce-
dures and helped me to bear up; the many
special nurses and medical staff at Toronto
General, Princess Margaret, and Women's
College hospitals of Toronto; the radiology
department and fundraising staff of the Arnot
Ogden Medical Center in Elmira, New York;
and the list goes on.

The National Ovarian Cancer Association,
through their connections and many volunteers, including my design and editorial team,
made this enterprise possible.

I am so very grateful to be here still. The fact
that I am, I believe, is a tribute to you all!

Foreword

I first met Dr. Annie Smith when she was referred to me with a probable diagnosis of ovarian cancer. A tall, fit woman with piercing blue eyes shook my hand firmly and announced that she had jogged the approximately eight blocks from her apartment in downtown Toronto to my office at Princess Margaret Hospital. At the time, I remember thinking that her choice of transportation was a little unusual. I did not yet understand Annie Smith's spirit or sense of humour.

That spirit and sense of humour emerged again in the operating room the following week. After Annie was asleep, the surgical team discovered that she had taped two chocolate bars to her abdomen, along with a message from a little bear, offering us a snack if we needed it to help us through the surgery.

That wasn't the only time Annie Smith got my attention with chocolate. When I returned to my office from Easter break a couple of months after first meeting Annie, I discovered chocolate eggs everywhere. She had managed to get into my office, where she hid Easter eggs in my lab coat, on books, in drawers, on the edges of picture frames — and in places I discovered only weeks later.

Whenever I saw Annie, she was drawing pictures of that little bear. Those pictures told her story about cancer, conveying without words what she went through. Even during her chemotherapy treatments, when she had to be hospitalized to control her side effects, she maintained her sense of humour and vitality, somehow mustering the energy to draw bears on the whiteboard in front of the nursing station to let the nurses know she was there. These pictures became conversation pieces around our ward and within the hospital.

Annie often spoke about writing a book about her experiences with cancer, using the bear to help her tell the story. I thought it was an interesting idea, but I didn't see how it would ever work.

My opinion changed dramatically, however, when I saw Annie give a presentation to a group of oncology nurses from across the United States. I sat mesmerized as she told her story through pictures of the bear. I found myself crying and laughing at the same time — and I realized what an immense gift she had in her ability to tell her story directly and sensitively, helping the audience relax and listen through her humour.

I wasn't the only one in awe that day. At the end of her talk, all two hundred people in the audience leapt to their feet to applaud not only a brilliant presentation on ovarian cancer, but also a woman with a unique gift for storytelling. Annie made us laugh and cry. But, in many ways, she also taught us — highly educated doctors, nurses, and health care workers — about ovarian cancer and its effects on women. For the most part, medical professionals see how illness affects our patients through our own eyes. Annie showed us ovarian cancer through *her* eyes, and in doing so gave us a radically different, and immensely valuable, perspective.

Yes, this book has many humorous stories and pictures. But it also tells a real story about a very serious disease. Annie holds nothing back. *Bearing Up with Cancer* will help people with cancer and their families understand and cope with this disease. It will also help health care providers better understand what our patients really experience.

Ovarian cancer affects approximately 2,500 Canadian women each year (25,000 women in the United States); roughly 60 per cent of women diagnosed will die from this very difficult disease. Improvements in treatment, however, continue to provide greater opportunities for remission. Developing genomic research will enhance our ability to understand why some women respond to treatment while others don't. At Princess Margaret Hospital, we hope to use these new technologies to help us better understand, prevent, and treat ovarian cancer.

Profits from the sale of this book will go to ovarian cancer research. With *Bearing Up*,

Annie has figured out a way to help people currently affected by ovarian cancer and — through research — those who will be affected by it in the future.

Annie Smith has helped me better understand what it is like to have cancer. She has inspired me to better understand my patient's needs, and to continue to try to find answers to the conundrum of ovarian cancer. Thank you, Annie, for helping me and so many others by sharing your story in *Bearing Up with Cancer*.

Dr. Barry Rosen, MD, FRCSC
Academic Chief, Division of Gynecologic Oncology,
Department of Obstetrics and Gynecology,
University of Toronto

Prologue

I'm not really a bear! I'm many things: an
artist, a teacher, a doctor of philosophy,
an author and lecturer, a sister and daughter,
a friend and colleague, a tennis player and
a sailor … and a woman who has lived with
cancer for nearly two decades. I've been
drawing my signature bear since childhood.
Over the last three years, I've drawn it as a
stand-in for me on my journey with this
disease. The bear has expressed my pain and
frustrations, my hopes and my joys. If you are
also coping with this disease, I hope that it
may be a comfort to you and your family
and friends.

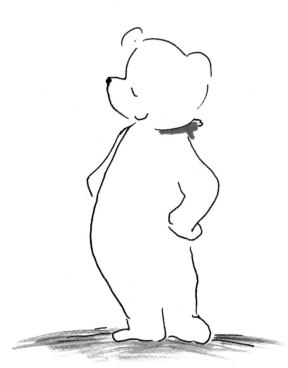

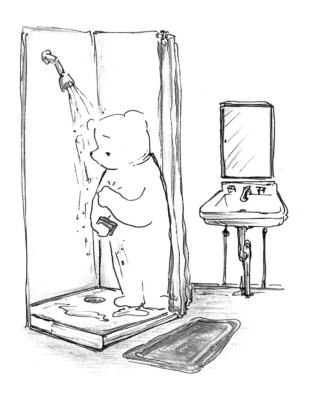

Chapter 1: In Which the Bear Finds a Lump

My cancer began in 1984, when I was forty-four years old. In the shower one morning, I felt a small lump in my right breast. So I went to the doctor. A specialist biopsied the nodule. I was told that if I didn't hear anything, all was fine.

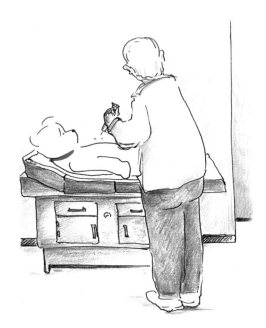

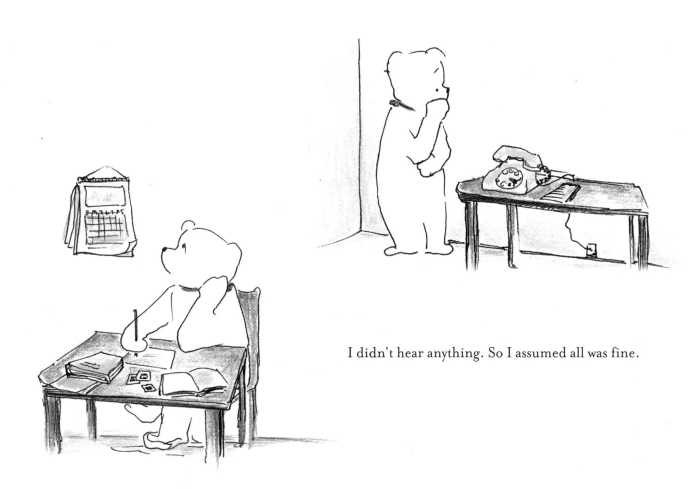

I didn't hear anything. So I assumed all was fine.

I got on with my teaching — art history and drawing and painting — and administering my unique undergraduate Art and Art History Program, offered collaboratively by the University of Toronto at Mississauga and Sheridan College in Oakville, Ontario.

A year passed.

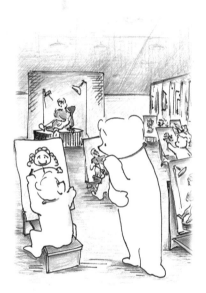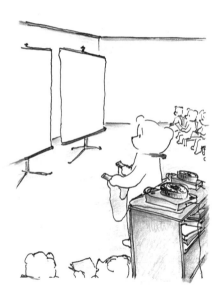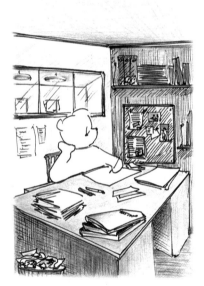

year off, free to pursue research, work on special projects, and play!

But I still had that lump. In fact, it seemed slightly larger. So I went back to the specialist to check that everything was indeed fine.

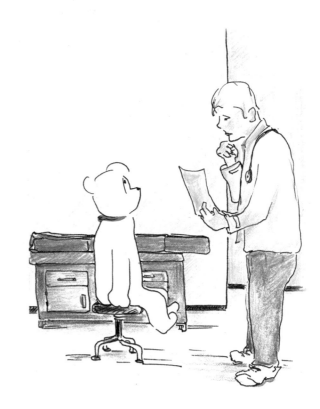

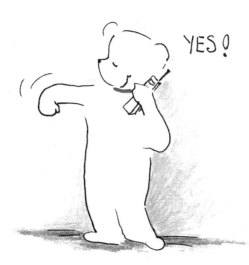

YES!

In the spring of 1986, I was awarded a sabbatical for the following academic year. How exciting! After twenty-plus years of teaching, I had my first opportunity for a

But all was not fine. The results of the biopsy were not in my file. They had been misplaced. Within days, I was scheduled for a lumpectomy.

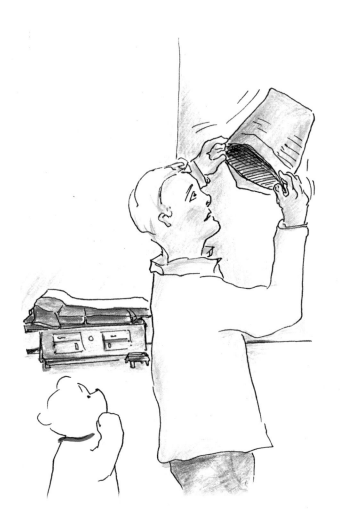

Chapter 2: In Which the Bear Has the First of Many Operations

That operation went well. It was a day-patient procedure. Waiting in the chilly operating room, I tried to entertain the surgeon with jokes: "Did you hear the one about the rope that walked into the bar? The bartender asked, 'Hey are you a rope?' 'No,' said the rope, 'I'm a frayed knot.'" Clearly, the drugs were beginning to take effect. Thankfully, I was soon in la-la land and could tell no more bad jokes.

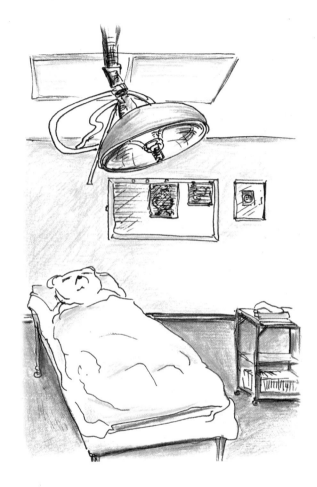

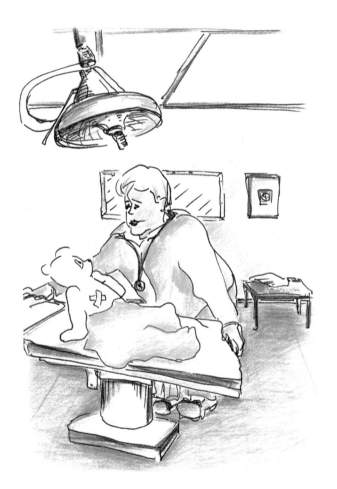

When I awoke in recovery, the surgeon reported that he had successfully removed a tumour and cancerous tissues from my breast. That was the good news. The less good news was that he had found small cancerous "nests" of cells located centrally beneath the nipple. He'd have to remove the entire breast — a mastectomy — the next morning.

The news hit like a ton of bricks. This was
big. Still, I tried to be cool about it. Since
they'd misplaced the biopsy a year before,
I asked the surgeon to please make sure that
they hadn't perhaps mistaken my nodules
for those of another patient. He smiled
and said he'd go double-check.

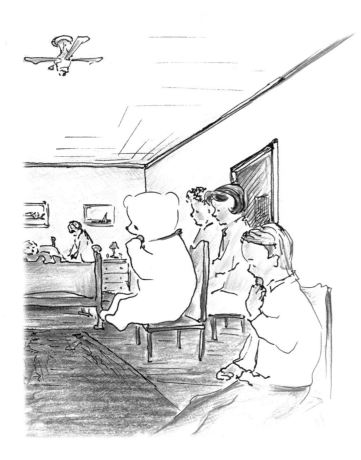

Lying there amidst others on stretchers in the recovery room, visions of my parents came to me. Both my parents had been medical professionals: Dad was a doctor, a radiologist, and Mom a nurse. And Mom had died of ovarian cancer. I recalled her suffering. She was so very ill, and so very gracious and strong in her ability to accept the inevitability of death. She was in great pain by the time the minister was invited to our home to say prayers and offer communion to the immediate family. I remembered being convulsed by grief, hardly able to swallow that dry wafer. I choked on the thimbleful of wine. I tried to shut out the words of the minister. I simply couldn't find them comforting, nor could I accept the approaching loss of my Mom.

As I lay on the stretcher, a couple of tears trickled from the corner of my right eye to my ear. A nurse brought me a tissue, and I regained my composure.

But the thoughts kept coming … Mom's illness … her death … should I be buried or cremated? My ear soon filled with tears once more.

My kind and gentle surgeon returned to say they had a room for me.

"Would you promise me something?" I asked. "Would you get a good night's rest and practise your stitches?"

I was an artist, I explained, and would appreciate an attractive job. He promised.

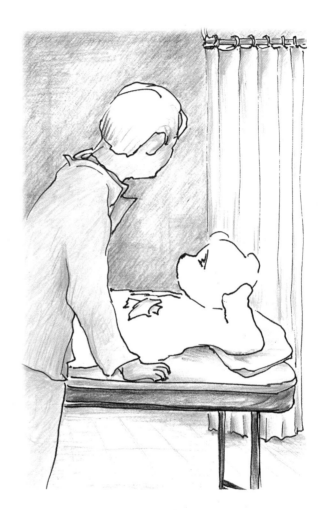

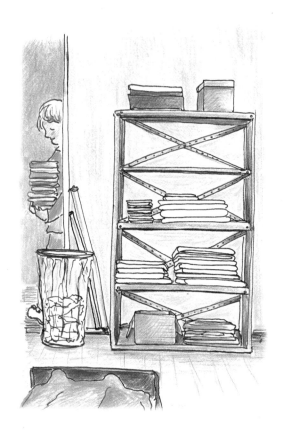

I was wheeled up to the isolation ward, the only floor where a room was available on short notice. I lay on a stretcher in the corridor while staff readied the room for me — it had been temporarily used as a storage area. I passed through double protective doors into a dismal, bare room with a view of a brick wall. It felt like a jail cell.

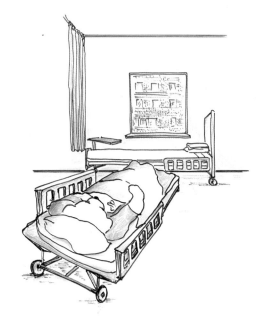

Once in that isolation ward, I began to think of all I had to do before the next day's operation: make arrangements with work for someone to cover my courses, notify friends and family, reschedule appointments. I had booked off only a couple days from work. I needed permission to leave the hospital, and bargained with the surgeon to let me leave:

"I'll return by five a.m."

"Let's say five p.m."

"How about midnight?"

"Six this evening!"

"Eleven!"

"Eight."

"Ten o'clock?"

"All right, ten o'clock."

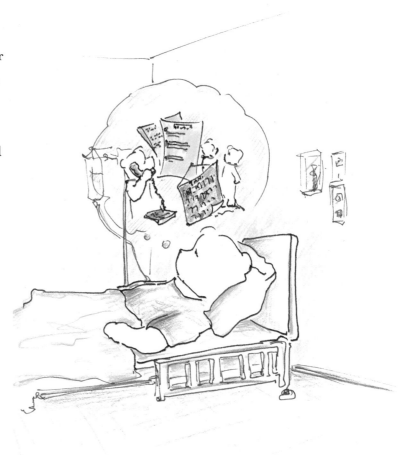

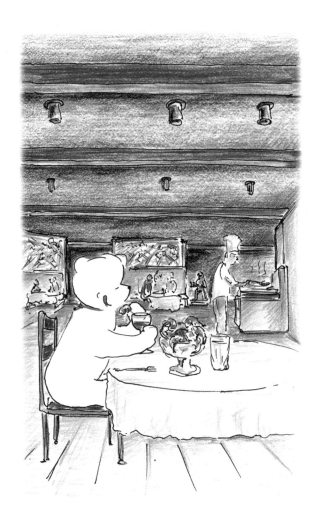

Sprung from my cell, I rushed from the hospital. I treated myself to a small but elegant bite in the Grill Room of the Windsor Arms Hotel's Three Small Rooms restaurant, across the street from my apartment. I ordered a shrimp cocktail and a glass of red wine, and I enjoyed them both immensely: I hadn't eaten since before the lumpectomy, and I wanted some fortification. By eight o'clock I had completed my various tasks. Lying on my bed, I listened over and over to Maria Callas sing an aria from my favourite part of Donizetti's *Lucia di Lammermoor*. I didn't know it at the time, but my choice of music was appropriate. Lucia's line "*Gioia diviene il pianto*" means "My sadness becomes joy."

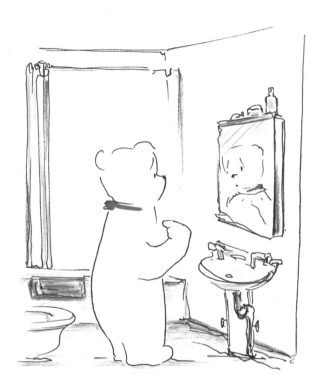

I looked in the mirror before I left.

"But you look so healthy," I said to my reflection. "How could you have cancer?"

By ten o'clock, I was back at the hospital, where I discovered that the nurses had bets on whether "Dr. Smith" would return by her deadline.

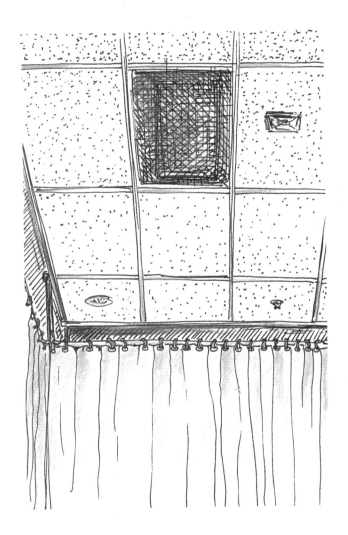

Chapter 3: In Which the Bear Studies Ceilings

I settled into my room and stared at the ceiling. My studies of ceilings had begun. So many ceilings! I have lain on my back and stared at ceilings from hospital beds, from gurneys outside operating rooms, from narrow tables in ultrasound and scanning rooms, from cots in doctors' examining rooms. Always, everywhere, the ceilings are the same, and they are boring: pockmarked, white panels held in place by strips of metal. Oh, of course they vary: some panels are stained. Some are chewed at the corners. Some are missing. Some boast air vents, sprinkler devices, lights.

But they are always, always boring. I long to bring them to life, to colour them, write on them, reproduce images from art history on them. No one who is ill — or who is healthy, for that matter — should be forced to stare at boring ceilings for hours on end.

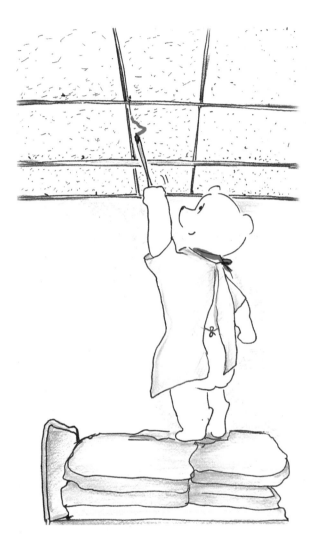

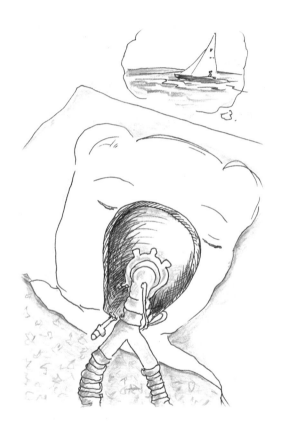

Chapter 4: In Which the Bear Has a Second Operation

The next morning, at six o'clock, I was wheeled into the operating room for my second surgery within twenty-four hours. This time, there were no bad jokes, although I did remind my surgeon of his promise about my stitches.

Recovery from the mastectomy wasn't as easy as the previous day's surgery. I awoke with tubes protruding from my chest – drains, the nurses told me. I was surprised to find that I couldn't raise my right arm: the muscles had been cut. Two general anesthetics within as many days left my voice box numbed and my internal system in disarray. My hospital stay lasted much longer than I expected it would, mostly because I never seemed to stop draining. The hemo-vac, an older model, kept clogging. I figured out how to take it apart, clean it, and reconnect it, much to the admiration of the nursing staff, who said things like, "Good thing you're a doctor and can fix these things." I didn't tell them I was a doctor of philosophy.

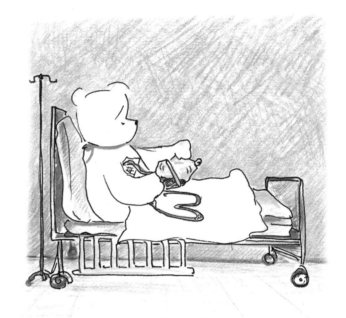

Chapter 5: In Which the Bear Is Scanned

Two days after my mastectomy, I began my
crash course in scans. Aside from a couple
of X-rays, I knew little of the world of ultrasounds, bone scans, CAT scans, and the like.
As the daughter of a radiologist, I suppose I
should have absorbed a bit more information
over the years. In fact, my birth announce-
ment had consisted of two images: one an
X-ray of me in the womb, the second of Dad,
the radiologist, wearing a mask and holding
me, newly born, in his arms. I had always
loved hanging around in the X-ray department with my dad, looking at the images.

Sitting in a wheelchair, hugging the
corridor wall outside the diagnostic rooms,
I was cold and lonely.

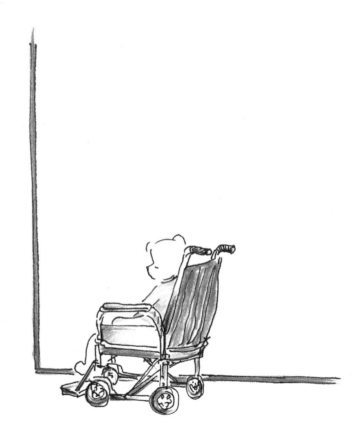

As my wait extended, however, my
loneliness diminished as the corridor filled
with other patients abandoned in their
chairs, waiting for their turns. I learned to
parallel park, and got quite good at reverse.
I even tried my hand at wheelchair wheelies.

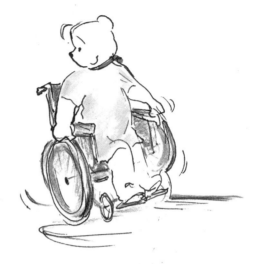

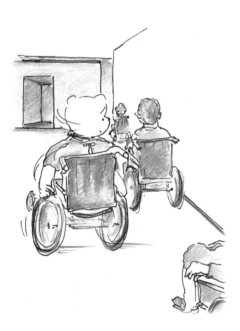

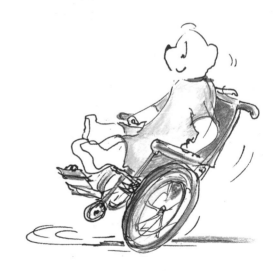

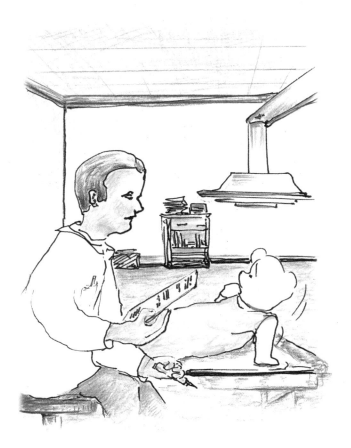

Finally, my turn arrived. The technician explained the procedure. Then, looking at my chart, he did a double take.

"How old are you?" he demanded.

"How old do you think I am?" I countered.

"Well, I'm not sure, but the Annie Smith on this chart is ninety-two years old!" he answered.

"Whatever gave you your first clue that she wasn't me?" I asked, relieved that at least this time the chart mix-up had been caught in time.

I was quickly disillusioned. The technician slathered me with a warm, gooey gel that soon turned clammy cold, and pummelled me with a plastic wand, which she pressed deep into various regions of my abdomen. I must have been a model patient, because she asked if her students could practise on me. Of course, I said, happy to be of help. One by one, they located the pancreas, the portal vein, and the "Playboy bunny": the hepatic veins and vena cava that together look like Hugh Hefner's mascot. I was good training ground for the class, but I emerged quite sore, and happy to return to my room.

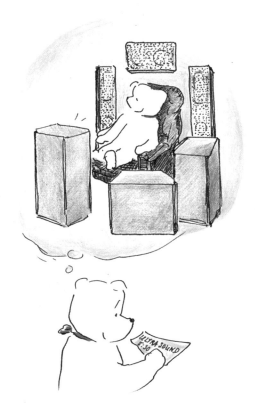

Next came the ultrasound. I envisioned myself embraced by the latest in audio science technology, perhaps enveloped in Dolby Stereo Surround Sound.

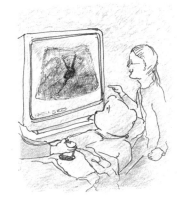

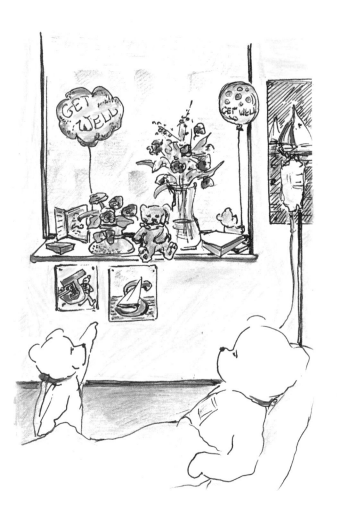

And my room! What a change from the dismal jail cell I'd slept in my first night at the hospital! The room was transformed: now aglow with flowers, posters, balloons, cards, and, of course, bears. Students and colleagues, friends and family, buoyed my spirits with joyful gifts and wishes. New staff, with their protective booties and gowns and caps and gloves, started in pleasant surprise upon entering my happy greenhouse.

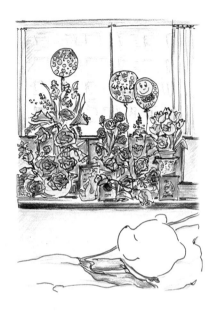

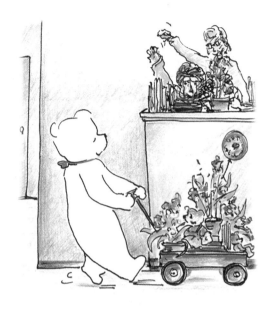

A handsome, tall Afro-Canadian, a member of the cleaning staff, broke into a wide grin as he slowly looked around. "Naaaiiice rooooooommm!" he said. In contrast, his colleague, a short Hungarian woman, took one look at all the plants and flowers and dashed to open the windows and remove the flora. "Aire, aire!" she cried. "Too many flores are eating all oxygen!"

Two weeks later, the tubes were removed, and I was released from the hospital. The fluids, however, continued to build up. For days following, I returned to the surgeon's office to have them drained.

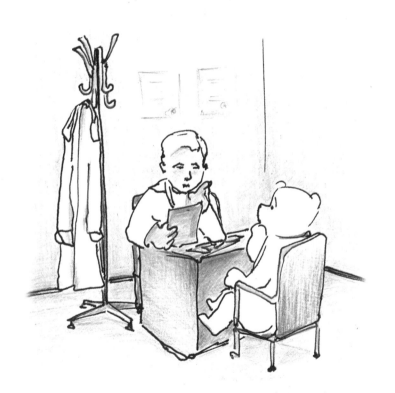

Chapter 6: In Which the Bear Attends Support Group, with Dubious Results

My prognosis was guardedly optimistic. The cancer had not spread to the lymph nodes, and I would not need chemotherapy. The surgeon asked if I would be willing to join a support group for those experiencing cancer.

"I don't think it'll be necessary," I said.

He told me he thought I would be good for the others in the group.

The support group had met once before I joined. As I walked into the room for my first session, I glanced at the people who had arrived before me. Some looked terribly ill, while others had the telltale look — little or no hair, emaciated, fatigued, skin grey or tinged yellow from jaundice — of people undergoing chemotherapy. And then there were a few like me, who sported the slightly weak, post-surgical look.

As the session began, I sat down beside a woman who was taking attendance.

"And who are you?" she whispered.

I glanced at the list and quietly pointed to my name.

"Fine," she said. She didn't make any mark in her attendance book. I noticed, however, that other names above mine had marks in the boxes beside them.

"What are those X's for?" I whispered.

"Oh," she replied, "they died."

"But I'm next on the list," I said, in mock horror.

"Oh, no—" she said, flustered by my response.

"Just a joke," I said. Obviously she didn't appreciate my sense of humour. Thus, I learned — and failed — my first lesson about support groups: don't make jokes. Especially not jokes about death.

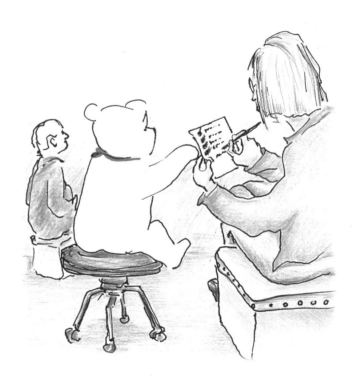

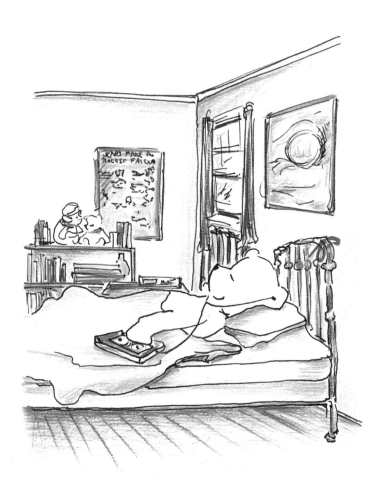

At the end of the session, the doctor gave me three meditation tapes, and instructed me to listen to them in the order prescribed.

Now, these were great. The voice on the tape was so mesmerizing as it instructed me to "Find a comfortable place to relax where you won't be disturbed ..." that I soon needed to hear only "Find a com—" and I was asleep.

"And how did you find the tapes?" the doctor asked at the next session.

"They're terrific!" I replied. "I'm asleep before the voice completes the first instruction!"

"Well, that's wrong!" he reprimanded me. "You aren't supposed to sleep, you're supposed to meditate. Don't you know the difference between relaxation, sleep, and meditation?"

Obviously, I had failed my second lesson.

At another session, we were each given a sheet of little green dots to take home and stick to surfaces as reminders to think positively about our battles with cancer. I was already pretty positive. Rather than clutter up my small apartment with little green dots, therefore, I used them on student files. And thus I failed my third lesson about support groups: follow instructions.

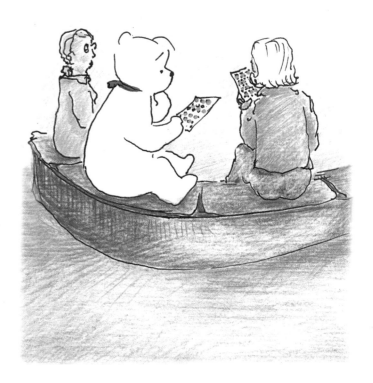

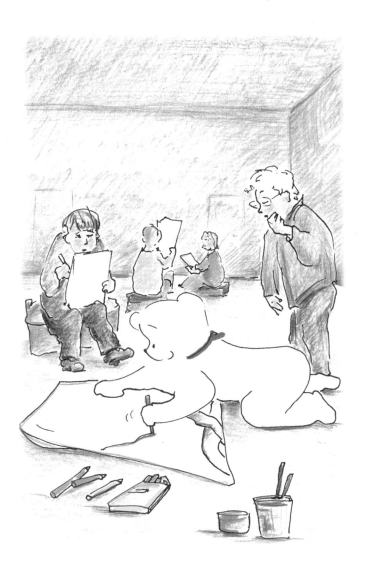

My next session began with the distribution of paper, crayons, markers, scissors, and the instructions to "visualize our cancer and draw how we would fight that battle."

What a great assignment! I set about visualizing the cancer cells as mean little gremlins marching through a maze of tangled blood vessels. The video game Pac-Man was popular at that time, so I drew teams of Pac-Man–like soldiers forming wedges and blockades and moving in on the cancer gremlins. Completely absorbed in my drawing, I didn't realize that the doctor was standing at my side, studying the images on my paper.

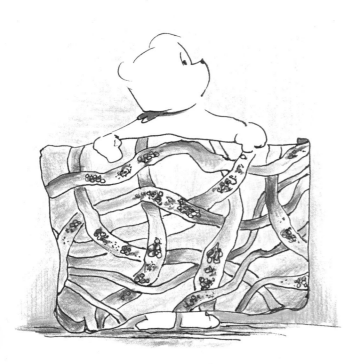

"What's this?" he asked.

With great detail and enthusiasm, I began explaining how the army was marching in on the cancer gremlins—

"This is supposed to be serious," the doctor interrupted.

"I am serious," I replied.

And with failed lesson Number 4, I stopped attending the support group.

Chapter 7: In Which the Bear Eats a Macrobiotic Diet

A little while after I stopped going to the support group, a friend who had recently experienced breast cancer brought me some delicious soup and homemade hummus, and shared a magazine that was devoted to an Asian doctor's theories on macrobiotic dietary approaches to fighting cancer. The doctor spoke of sushihane (seaweed), shitake mushrooms, udon (noodles), edamame (soy beans), and tofu (which, when I first heard its name, I thought was "toe food" — much like "finger food," I guessed). I loved the soup and the hummus and purchased a book on macrobiotic cooking.

The first recipe I chose called for Chinese radish, ginger, tahini, and tofu. I mixed the ingredients together and sampled my creation. Something was missing. I added more ginger, tasted, added a bit more, tasted, and … whoops, too much ginger. I countered the ginger with tofu, and tasted … too bland. No problem, I thought, I'll add more radish. I tasted yet again … too strong of radish. Well, more tahini should do the trick …

On and on I went until I had filled a huge pot with colourless — and quite tasteless — healthy stuff. Boring! A little like those ceiling panels. My initial enthusiasm for macrobiotic cooking soon waned.

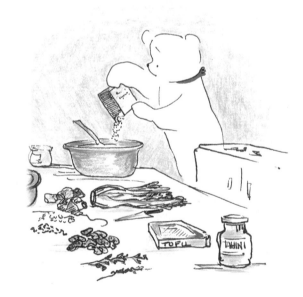

Chapter 8: In Which the Bear Finds, and Loses, a Prosthesis

When my mastectomy scars had healed suffi-
ciently, I was sent to a prosthesis salon to be
fitted with a new right breast. My breasts were
never very big, and I really had no desire for
a prosthesis: the idea of anything artificial
didn't appeal to me. But my doctors told me
that if I didn't replace the right breast I would
likely develop back problems because of the
imbalance. So I complied.

I hated the thing! It *was* artificial, even
though the consistency felt vaguely flesh-like
and it boasted the suggestion of a nipple.
It was heavy, far heavier than my real breast,
I thought. Oh no, I was told, I simply had no
idea how weighty flesh is.

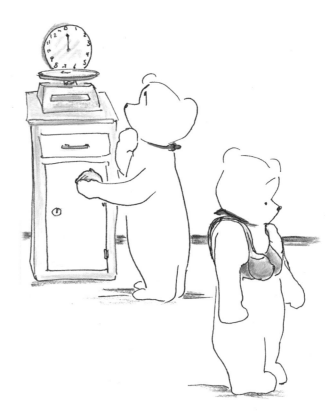

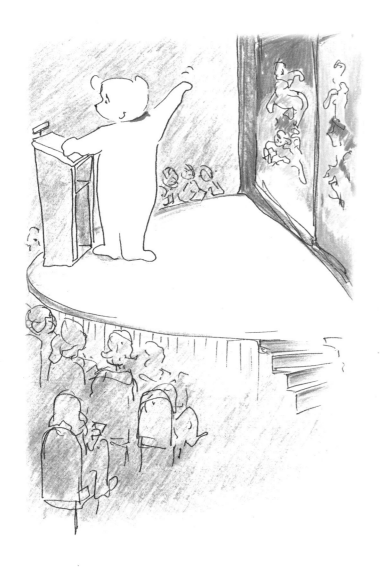

I didn't wear the prosthesis playing tennis, but I did comply with the doctor's recommendations and dutifully wore it during my public appearances. That is, I wore it for a few years.

And then there was the day I gave a lecture at a conference of about 350 art educators from across Canada. I always lectured with a double projection of slides. Someone had left a pencil on the podium, and somehow, while manipulating the remote controls for the slides, I knocked the pencil off.

Casually, I leaned down to pick it up. And wouldn't you know, that prosthesis just slipped out and bounced across the stage. Relieved it didn't bounce right off the stage, I picked up both pencil and prosthesis, slipped the latter back into my bra, and muttered, "God, I'm glad the other one is attached!" I went right on with the lecture. I'm sure the audience members who saw what happened were initially horrified, but in the end we laughed together.

From that day forward, I have never worn the prosthesis. My back is fine. And one of my students finally put the artificial right breast to good use when she used it in an art project.

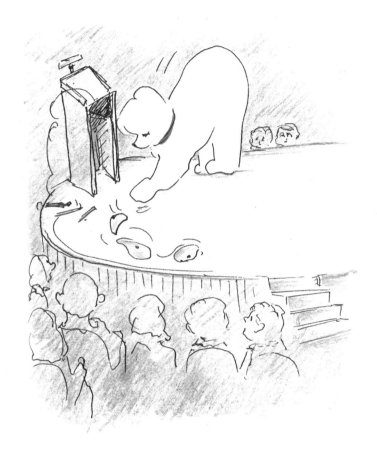

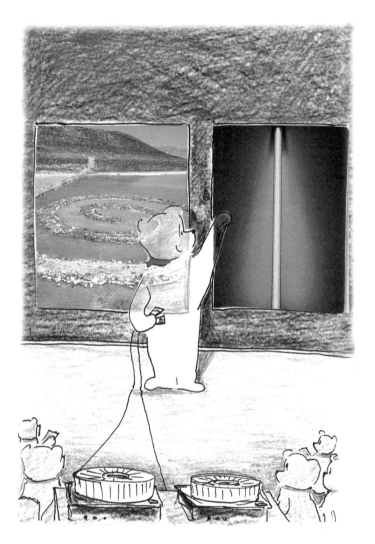

Chapter 9: In Which the Bear Is Awarded Another Sabbatical

Soon I was healed and back in full flight, teaching and leading the Art and Art History Program to new challenges, while lecturing nationally and internationally. In 1993, I published my first book, *Getting into Art History*. Visits to the doctors indicated that I was cancer-free. My only complaint was that I felt tired, which I figured was due to a heavy workload and getting older.

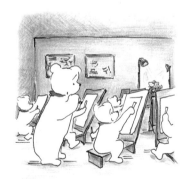

In 1994, however, a curious nodule developed within my right chest wall, likely a growth related to the breast cancer and caused by a wayward cell that had escaped during the operations. The nodule was surgically removed. It was cancerous, but there was no follow-up chemotherapy or radiation.

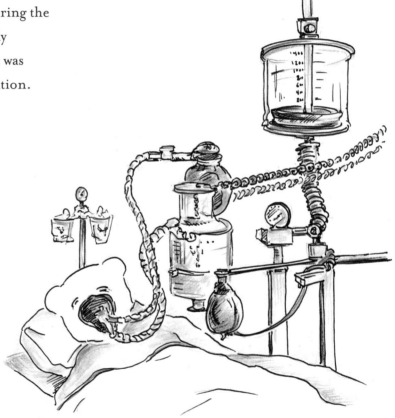

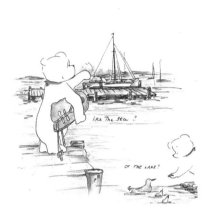

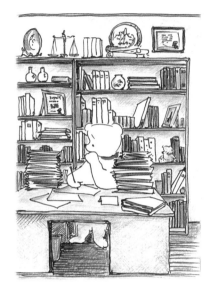

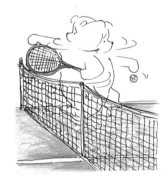

I was back on track after a short leave of absence, carrying on with administration, lecturing, sailing, tennis, and living the life of a regular busy being. To paraphrase John Lennon, life is what happens while you're busy making other plans.

Life was happening. All seemed to be going well.

And then, in June 1998, I was awarded another sabbatical. Another opportunity to work and research and read and travel and write and play — or so I thought.

I really should have known. I will never take another sabbatical — I think I must be allergic to them.

Not long after getting the sabbatical news, I felt a hard mass in the lower left quadrant of my abdomen. So back I went to the doctor. I drew a bear indicating the position of the mass and asked where the ovaries were located.

"Much higher than that," she replied. "Relax and have a great sabbatical."

And I was out the door to do just that.

We had both been too casual. My mom's death from ovarian cancer was in the back of my mind, but I was anxious to move forward with my various projects, so I didn't dwell much on this latest aberration.

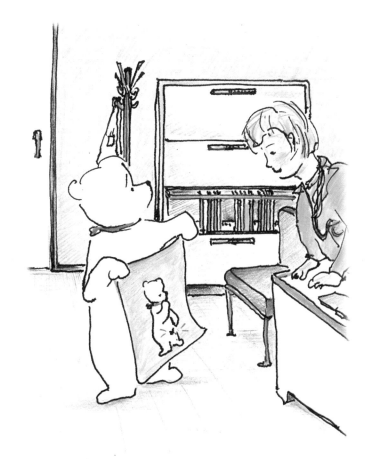

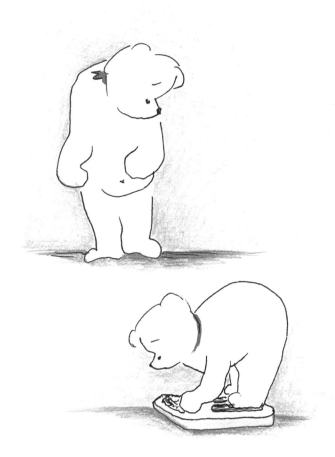

Chapter 10: In Which New Gremlins Surface

By February of 1999, I was well into my sabbatical year, involved in a project of videotaping interviews with Canadian women artists and preparing for a keynote speech for a conference of art teachers in British Columbia. In the middle of it all, that mysterious mass in my abdomen seemed to go on a rampage. It was suddenly larger and weightier. I felt bloated. I also noticed that I was gaining weight. My doctor couldn't see me until the end of March, however, so I figured I would get it checked out once I returned from my conference.

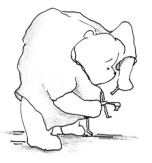

A stress fracture in my right hand a few days before I was to leave for Vancouver, however, meant that I saw the doctor earlier. There, I inquired once more about my mysterious mass. Within what seemed like minutes, I had struggled my way into yet another blue hospital gown and found myself covered with gooey gel and staring at yet another boring ceiling as an ultrasound technician prodded my belly with her wand. I held a mirror in my hand so I could see the ultrasound screen.

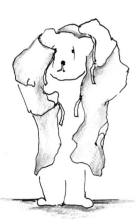

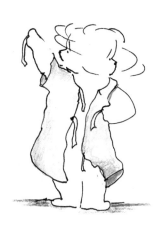

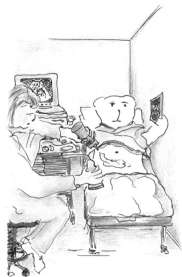

The technician called in a senior technician. The senior technician called in the radiologist. The radiologist called in a colleague, and they all engaged in professional discussions on the other side of the curtain. They made calls to arrange that I see my doctor — immediately.

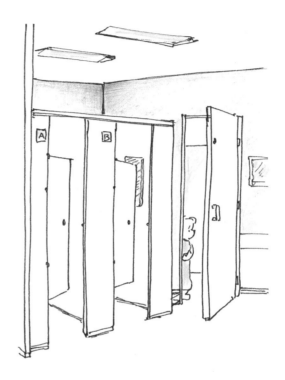

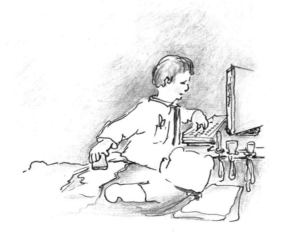

"Oh, boy," I thought. "I'm in deep trouble now."

Chapter 11: In Which the Bear Prepares for Surgery

"You know what it is?" asked my doctor.

"Yes," I replied. "I suspect it's ovarian cancer."

"So what's your schedule like?"

"I leave tomorrow morning to give the keynote speech at a conference in British Columbia."

"And you return when?"

"In late March?" I replied hopefully.

"Not a chance!" was her response. "More like immediately after the presentation! And if you have any discharge or experience any significant changes in your health, get to a Vancouver hospital right away. That tumour is large enough to rupture or cause unexpected and serious problems."

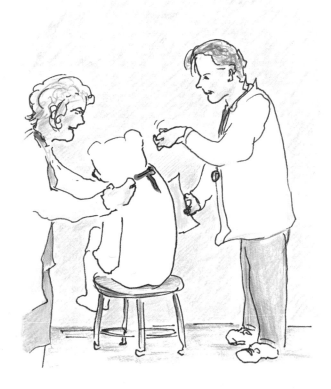

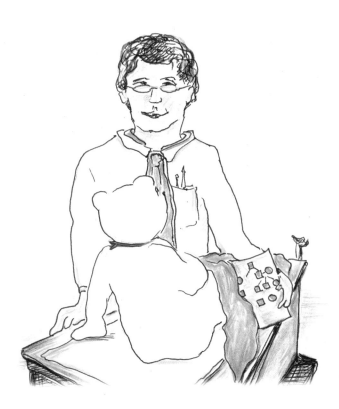

With that warning, I got on the plane. My lecture was successful, although I was somewhat apprehensive, what with all those warnings. I returned as instructed and met with the surgeon, a gynecological oncologist.

I liked him immediately. His name was Barry — a good sign. I chose to think of him as "Beary." He was right up my alley — he was even into art. He drew diagrams of my family tree, and he had visual charts on which he drew ovaries and approximated the location of my gremlins.

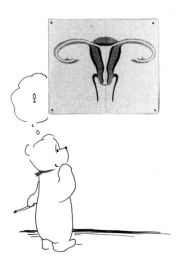

Every chance I get, I alter these ovarian charts, creating surreal images of bulls or deer. I make horns and antlers of fallopian tubes, and turn uteri into animal heads and noses.

The surgeon's explanations were succinct, his examination confirmed the gravity of the situation, and within an hour he had scheduled tests for the next day. He instructed me not to eat, gave me forms that would admit me to the hospital on Sunday, and promised to work me into his operating schedule on Monday.

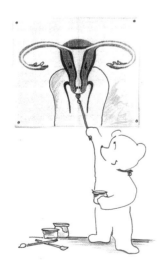

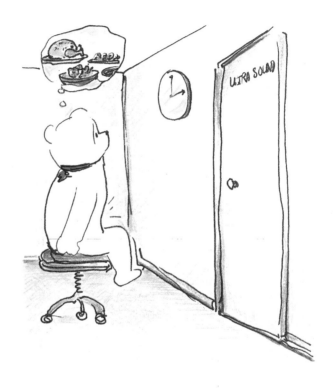

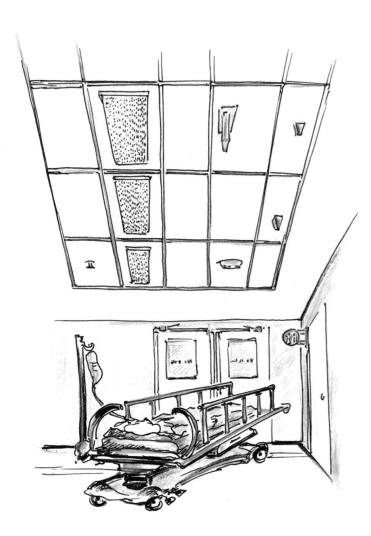

Chapter 12: In Which the Bear Prepares for Surgery – Again

Well, it didn't work. The Monday operation, that is. Sunday I was cleaned out internally, prepared mentally, and bedded down in another dull hospital room with a boring ceiling. Monday, with the IV in place, I waited and waited some more. I was more than ready to have those gremlins removed. So were my surgeon and his team. But late in the afternoon, the operating room police cancelled the procedure. They decided that the complex nature of the operation – a total abdominal hysterectomy and bilateral salpingo-oopherectomy, or the removal of my uterus, cervix, ovaries, and fallopian tubes – would throw off the schedule for all the subsequent operations that day.

I was disappointed. So was my special gynecological oncologist, but he resolved to work me in as soon as possible. I resolved not to have any solid foods so I wouldn't have to repeat the internal cleansing process. On Wednesday I was again admitted to the hospital. By Thursday morning I was feeling weak and awash — I'd been on a liquids-only diet for four days.

The hours passed slowly. I wheeled my IV stand around the perimeter of the surgical "holding room," drawing bears in the blank spaces on the boards where operation schedules were posted. There were bears on stretchers watching the clocks outside the operating room, bears lined up in hospital corridors with IVs in place, and bears preparing for the upcoming St. Patrick's Day. I drew a birthday card for Evan, the anesthetist.

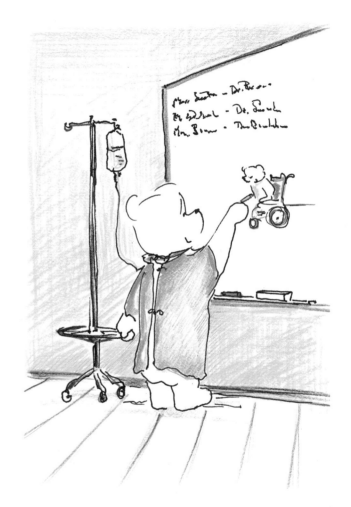

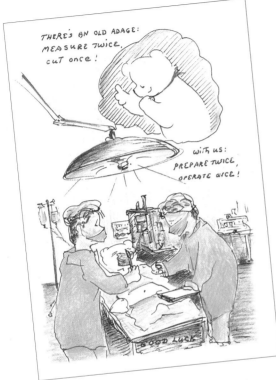

I also drew a message to my surgical team: "There's an old adage: measure twice, cut once. With us: prepare twice, operate once!" I taped it to my abdomen, along with two candy bars. Over that was my hospital gown and over that — by the time I finally got on the operating table at 1:30 that afternoon! — was a warm blanket.

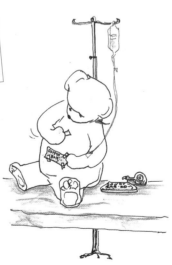

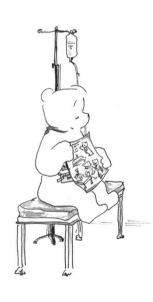

Monitors were placed up and down my sides. I stared at the complex array of machines and wondered when the surgical team would find the surprise. But I was out of it when they discovered the note and candy bars. Word has it I made quite a stir.

And so, we had indeed prepared twice, and operated once. But this operation was far more complex than the mastectomy. And so was my recovery.

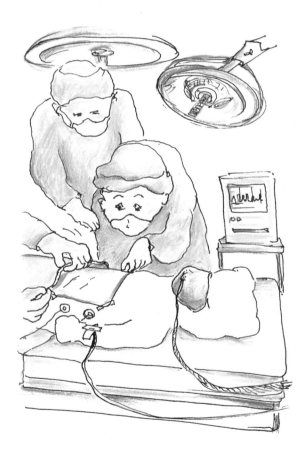

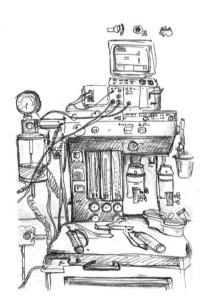

Chapter 13: In Which the Bear Has Little Fun

There were many surprises. The first was that, when I looked down at my swollen abdomen, I saw that the incision had been closed by a series of silver rings, much like those that adorn my students' noses, lips, ears, and navels, to mention only a few obvious places.

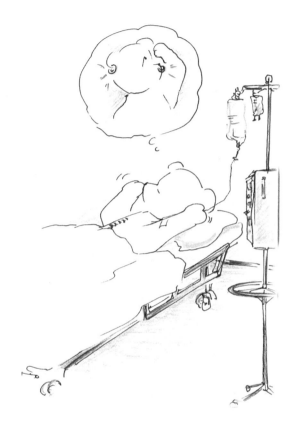

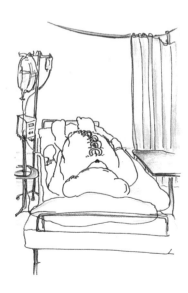

Whatever happened to stitches? I felt my ears and nose to make sure the surgeons hadn't played a trick on me. With a ring in my navel, however, I was part of the gang!

That incision was evidence of a major operation. The cancer, my surgeon told me later,
had spread to both ovaries, my uterus, my fallopian tubes, and my cervix. I also had deeply
situated pelvic lymph-node tumours that could
not be removed. They had gutted me. I was
pretty empty.

And I was pretty sick. In the first four days
there seemed to be only setbacks. Days passed
with me on a diet of ice chips and morphine —
even the pre-surgery all-liquid diet was beginning to look good. There were blood tests and
urine tests and transfusions. There were ultrasounds and X-rays and more scans. I had a high
fever that raged for almost two weeks. It was
accompanied by insomnia, severe headaches,
and vomiting.

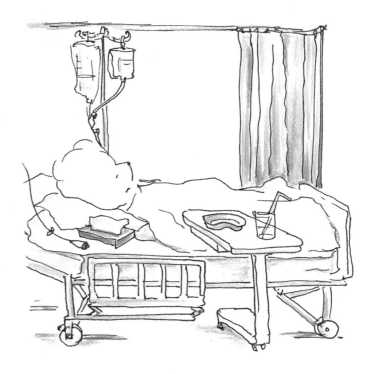

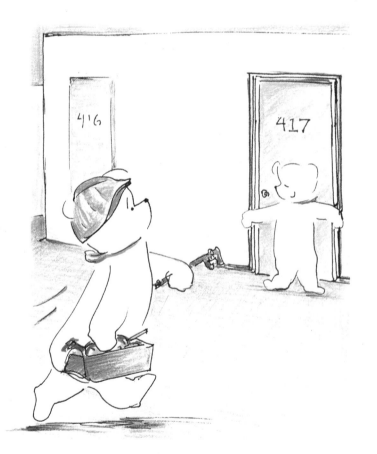

Every nurse who entered my room asked whether I had passed any gas. I hadn't, much to their disappointment, and my own.

On the fifth day, however, I thought I heard a small squeak and decided that indeed I had passed a little gas, so I drew an image of a hydro repairman, wrench and tool box in hand, racing down the corridor saying, "Quick, quick, I hear there is a small gas leak in room 417!" A little bear blocking the door replied, "Don't fix it, it's progress!" I took the drawing to the nurses at their station.

That accomplishment meant that I was finally allowed liquids. It took me three-quarters of an hour to swallow half a cup of warm water with lemon and two teaspoons of Jell-O. Then I threw up.

By evening, my blood pressure had risen, my temperature had risen, my pulse rate had risen, and I was vomiting violently. My abdomen was so distended that it reminded me of those horrific pictures of starving children with bloated bellies — but with rings.

On the sixth day, I hemorrhaged. Bloody liquids began to surge from my vagina, a discharge of peritoneal fluids. I looked — and felt — like the victim of an axe murderer. The loss of fluids was enormous. How could so much liquid come out the bottom when so little was going in the top?

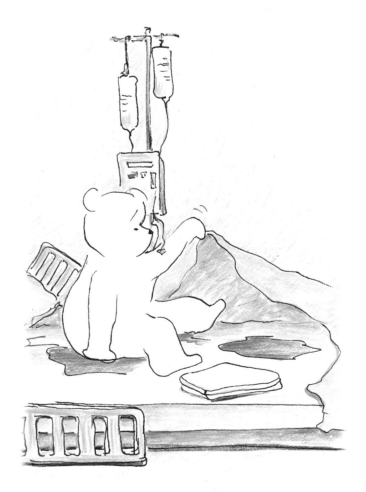

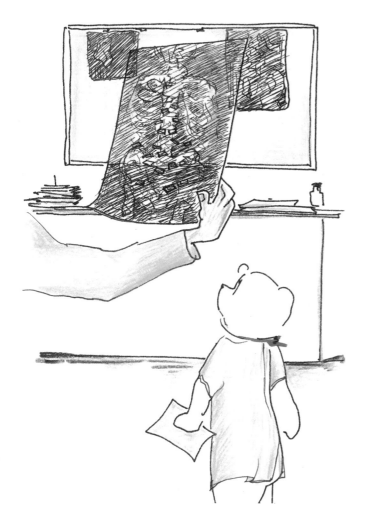

A series of excruciatingly painful internal examinations, ultrasounds, and X-rays checked me for internal bleeding, the accumulation of blood in the abdominal cavity, and possible bowel obstruction. I couldn't even stomach ice chips. I was miserable.

But friends and family called, sent flowers and cards, and gave me reading material and bears. A colleague treated me to a "therapeutic touch" session, in which a tall, lovely women hovered over me with healing hands that created a warmth, a magnetic field of sorts, around my body.

The nurses admonished me to keep using the incentive spirometer, a device designed to exercise the lungs and prevent a buildup of fluids. They also encouraged me to walk the halls. I would drag my IV pole as far as the operations schedule board just across from the nurses' station and draw a bear or two in the blank space that seemed always available in the board's lower right corner. Then I'd return to my den to rest and suck ice chips, which I was once again permitted.

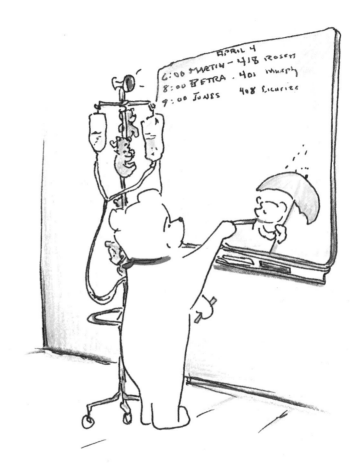

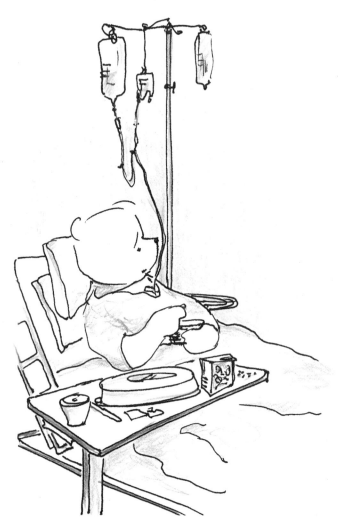

Several days later, the fever broke. I ate sixty-four individual Rice Krispies and a cracker. Food began to stay down. The tubes came out. I was given handfuls of literature on "Chemo and You."

Twenty-two days after the hospital ordeal
had begun, and twenty-two pounds lighter,
I went home. The skin on my legs sagged.
It looked like chicken skin! I felt as though
I had shrunk several inches: my muscles
drooped and my clothes dragged. Seeing my
reflection in store windows, I thought I
looked old, tired, thin, wrinkled, and sick!
And if that weren't enough, I was about to
experience chemotherapy.

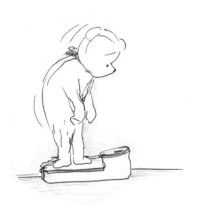

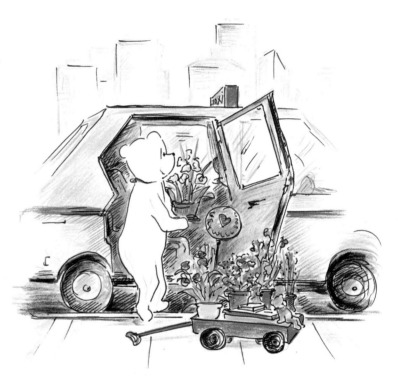

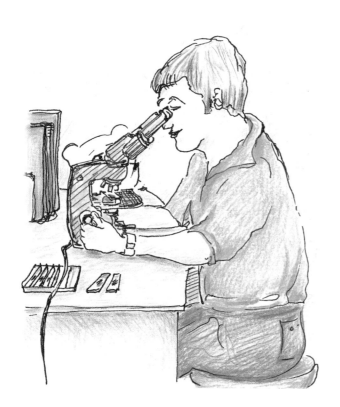

Chapter 14: In Which the Bear Encounters the Tumour Board

Chemotherapy following surgery has become standard practice in many cases in order to destroy the vagrant gremlin cells that might stray through blood vessels, looking for a new place to dwell. In my case, because of my inoperable pelvic tumours, it was imperative to follow surgery with chemotherapy treatment as soon as possible.

But what kind of treatment? The chemotherapy "cocktail" one receives depends upon the type of cancer one has — and there are many types of ovarian cancer. My pathology report, however, didn't give a clear answer as to which kind I had. The cellular imagery matched neither that of breast metastasis nor the typical ovarian expressions, so my case was presented to the famous "tumour board."

I envisioned a board covered with weird growths. Actually, the board was made up of pathologists, oncologists, microbiologists, and gynecological specialists, who gathered to review special problem cases. My doctor favoured the CAP chemotherapy series, which would, in effect, attack both breast and ovarian cancer cells. He suggested I discuss the decision with one of his colleagues, a senior oncologist at the hospital.

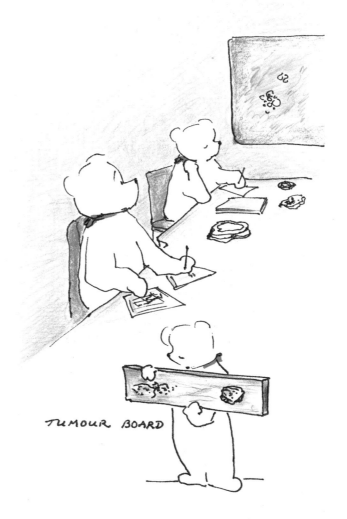

TUMOUR BOARD

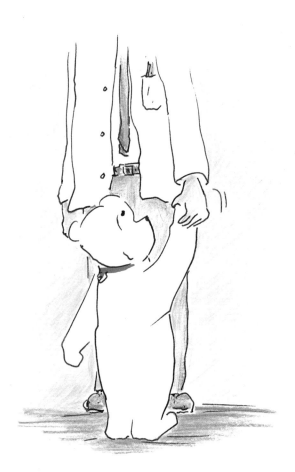

This specialist, a very tall, thoughtful, and soft-spoken gentleman, introduced himself. I stood, extended my hand, and said, "How do you do, Doctor, I've been dying to meet you! Well, er, I mean, perhaps that's a bad choice of words." When he told me he hoped to buy me more time, I immediately asked how much fifty years would cost! Sometimes you think to yourself, I can't believe I just *said* that.

Chapter 15: In Which the Bear Has Chemotherapy

My doctors and I agreed on the CAP series —
six monthly treatments of Cisplatin,
Adriamycin (a.k.a. the "Red Devil"), and
Cyclophosphamide. Together, they make for
a truly toxic cocktail, one so potent that it is
less favoured for current treatment. In fact,
my mother had gone through chemotherapy
with Cisplatin, but hadn't tolerated it at all
well. She died after her fourth treatment.

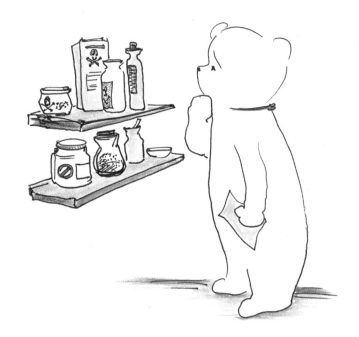

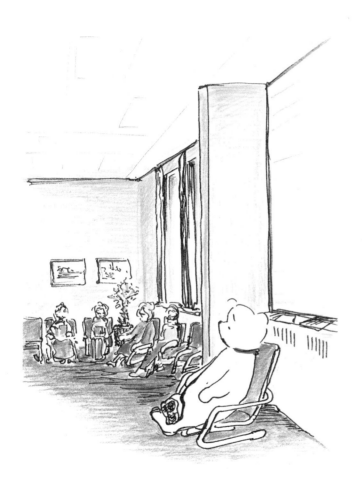

My brother flew in from the West, as did two friends from the Midwest, and we made a celebratory event of the first chemo. None of us knew what to expect or how I might react, so I prepared for everything and anything.

First I waited in the blood clinic, and then in the gynecological clinic for the results of the bloodwork and the gynecological oncologist's go-ahead for the chemo. That took most of the morning.

As I waited, I noticed constant announcements over the hospital PA system: "Would Mr. Stevenson please return to Day Care?" "Would Mrs. Kelly please return to Day Care?" I envisioned an unruly bunch of children behaving badly and tormenting their beleaguered caregivers, who finally called the parents back for assistance. Imagine my shock when my next instructions were to report to Day Care. What? Go there with all those nasty kids? I didn't think so.

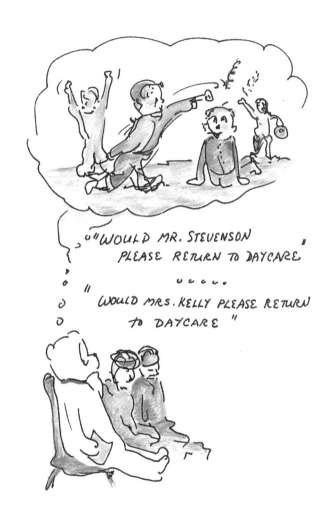

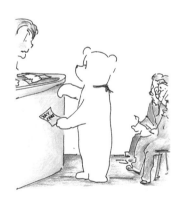

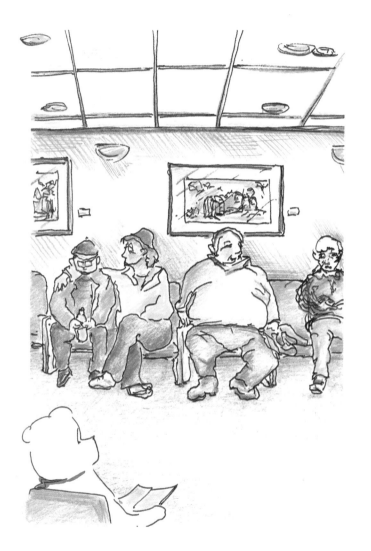

Day Care, however, turned out to have an altogether different meaning. There were no misbehaving children. In fact, there were no children at all. We were all adults, all cancer patients, all there for same-day chemotherapy treatment. We were young, old, male and female, of every nationality and ethnic persuasion, representing various stages of the havoc caused by cancer. Another long waiting period preceded my foray into the treatment centre itself.

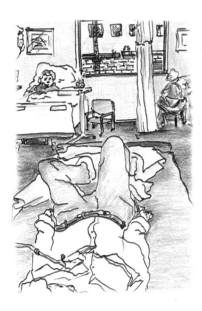

the various ill effects of the drugs, the steroids, the bags of liquid magnesium, and the various other chemicals required to supplement and balance individual needs. Regulatory machines on the IV poles bonged each time one of these bags emptied. The sound nauseated me. This was definitely not a happy place. I was glad to have my brother and friends with me.

The treatment centre was a long corridor lined with pink and green Naugahyde La-Z-Boy chairs interspersed with some beds and a few rooms that could be isolated. Every chair and bed was occupied. The pink and green colours made me feel sick, as did the bags upon vinyl bags of clear liquids. There were bags of saline solution, the toxic chemotherapy drugs, the "anti-anti's" that counteracted

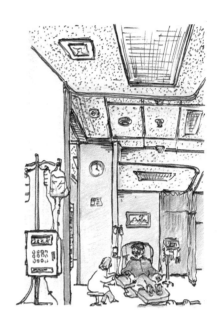

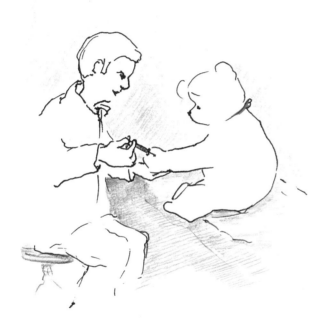

My Irish nurse carefully pushed the "Red Devil" into my vein, all the while informing us about the possible side effects. I was to keep drinking liquids to flush my system of the toxic chemicals. With each bathroom visit I became increasingly aware of the obnoxious odours caused by the drugs. I was soon sickened by the smell. I felt allergic to myself.

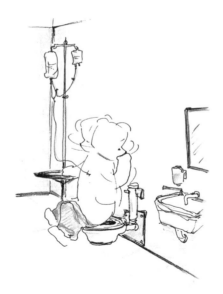

About five hours later, the session was
over. I was still walking, talking, and feeling
fairly normal — despite the periods during
which my body seemed to be burning up
from within, or my head split with aches,
or I burped and felt queasy, or my face
grew bright red and puffy. "Steroids," said
my nurse.

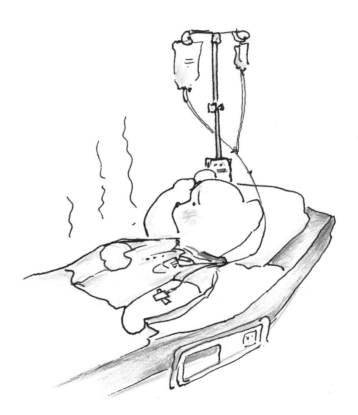

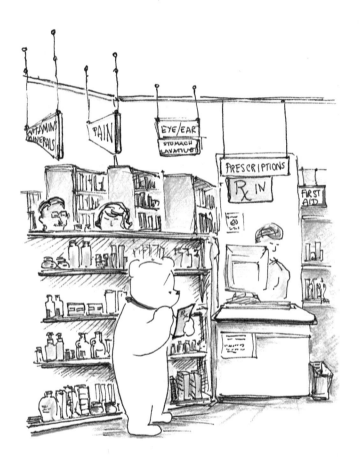

The pharmacy filled my prescriptions to counter the side effects of the chemo. I had headaches and nausea. The drugs to offset the headaches and the nausea caused insomnia and constipation. The drugs to offset the insomnia and the constipation caused extreme diarrhea. I bounced between drugs for about a week until my intestines began to settle down and a few foods started to appeal to me. I had made it through my first chemo.

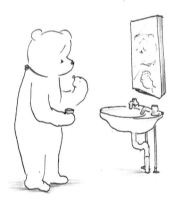

By the second week following chemo I was
ready to travel. Friends drove me to my old
barn on a lake where I had spent almost every
summer of my life.

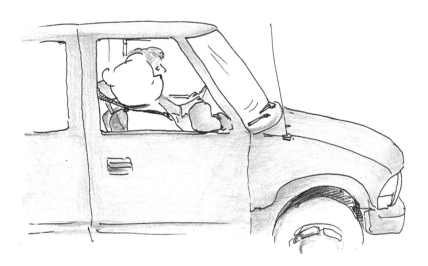

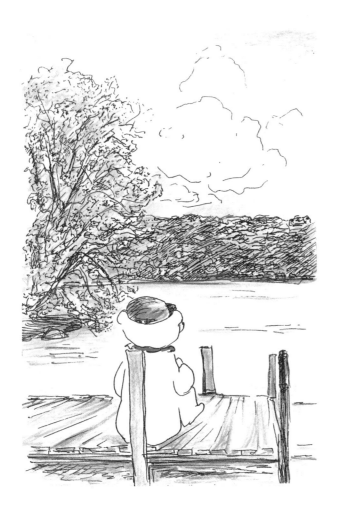

At the barn, I could stare at the water and sky and reflections, listen to birds and wind and waves, smell lilacs and fresh-cut grass, and relish the joys of nature. I was at my "healing place." I sat on the grass, pulling up a few dandelions and admiring their tenacity and will to survive. I took some courage from these little plants that seem to defy nature and push their way through solid rock. Although I was overwhelmed with fatigue and had little more than enough energy to sit on the lawn and pick dandelions, I was restored by the familiarity of place and sound.

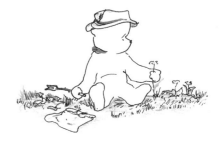

70

Chapter 16: In Which the Bear Has More Chemotherapy

Quickly, too quickly, a month passed. It was back to the hospital and back to waiting — in the blood clinic, the gynecological clinic, the Day Care, and the treatment centre.

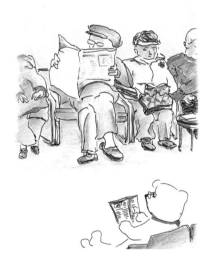

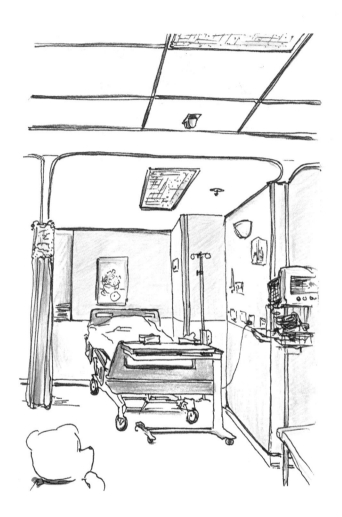

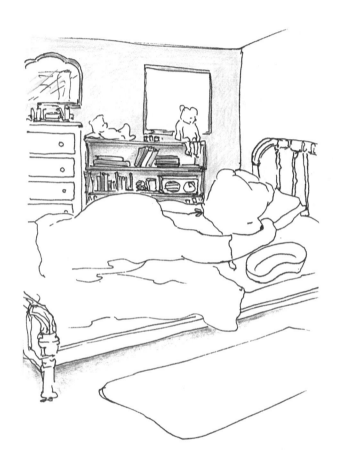

The way you tolerate your first chemo, I had been told, usually indicates how well you'll get through the remaining treatments. I hoped, therefore, that the second treatment would be as relatively uneventful as the first. But such was not the case. The second chemo truly undid me. Not long after returning to my apartment, I started to vomit. My temperature rose, my vision blurred, and waves of nausea and vomiting hit every twenty minutes or so. I was sick, sick, sick. I managed to contact the gynecologist on call at the hospital, who explained that she would rather not send me to emergency, where I would sit and wait forever. She suggested I try to get through the night on my own and go immediately to the clinic in the morning.

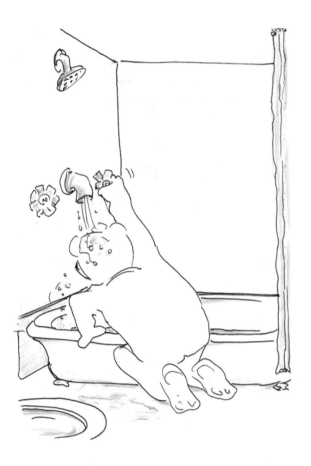

That night was frightening and unbearably long. When my head wasn't over the toilet, it was under the cold-water tap in an attempt to lower my raging fever.

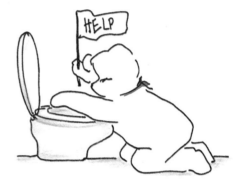

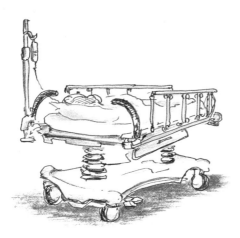

From that chemo on, I was transferred after treatment from Day Care to the gynecological floor, where I would spend several days being hydrated and "de-nauseated" intravenously. To this day I can't stand looking at a can of ginger ale.

When I entered the clinic the next morning, my own gynecological surgeon greeted me. "You really are sick, aren't you?" he said. I was immediately hospitalized so we could start running fluids to help protect my healthy parts from the ravages of the chemo.

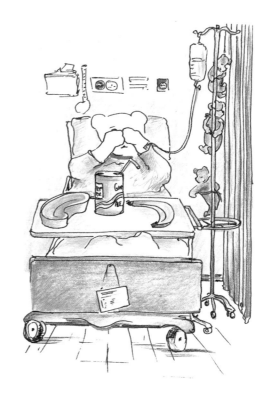

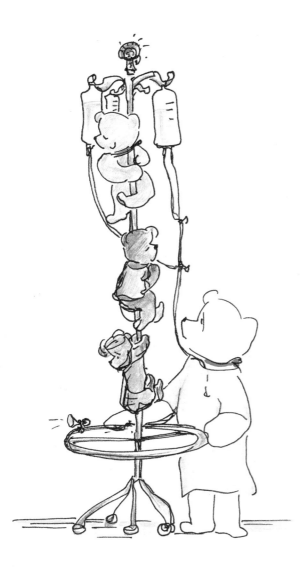

I prepared for my monthly hospital stay by packing a little bag with special accessories.

I attached bears to my IV pole, along with my battery-run blinking bike light and a small horn whose "beep-beep" was oddly reminiscent of the Roadrunner. I was no roadrunner, but when I did venture into the corridor for a short walk my rig attracted smiles and comments — and all the children visiting their sick elders. I felt like the Pied Piper of Ward 9 as I made my way through the corridors with my entourage of kids, stopping at the surgeons' operating schedule board to draw a "bear for the day" in one of the corners.

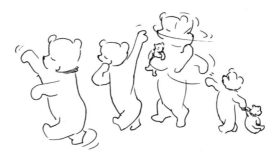

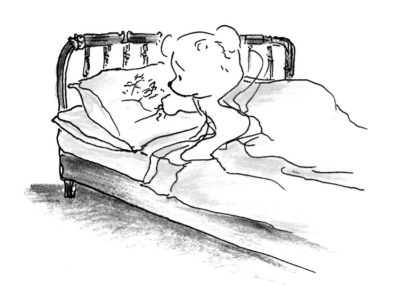

Chapter 17: In Which the Bear Loses Hair

Shortly after the third chemotherapy session, I awoke to find my pillow covered with hair. It was ugly, drifting into folds of sheets and blankets, catching in my eyes. I thought of the artist Méret Oppenheim's fur-lined cup, saucer, and spoon as I felt hairs in my mouth. I thought about cutting it all off, but I had a thick head of hair and wondered just how much I would actually lose. I decided to wait a bit.

My shedding was a true detriment to any social gathering. I don't see why anyone wanted to invite me to a party. With one nod of my head I could wipe out an entire cheese tray or ruin a perfectly good Scotch.

I hadn't realized that when you lose hair because of chemotherapy, you lose hair every place you have it: your nose, and ears, your armpits, legs, and — yes, everywhere! Now I know why we have hair in all those places — it's to keep the flaps from sticking together!

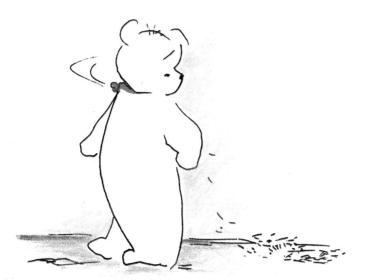

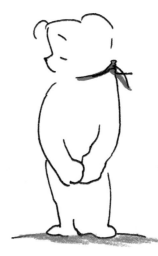

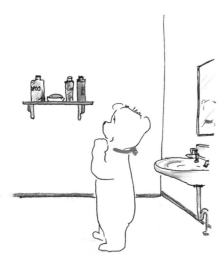

On the positive side, I suppose I saved money on shampoo and haircuts. And I learned to identify with balding men: when it rained, it felt like marbles bouncing off my head. I began to wear sporty caps to keep my head warm in the cold and cool in the heat. Even my tennis game improved, but that was mostly because there was so much static electricity in the bubble where I played in winter. The static caused what hair I had left to stand straight up. My opponents fell apart at the freakish hilarity of it all — and as they lost concentration, my score went up accordingly.

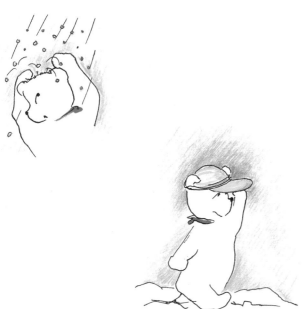

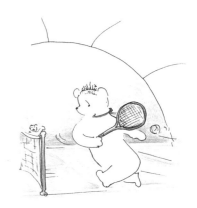

The wig salon was terrific fun. I wasn't sure I really wanted a wig. I knew the hair loss was temporary and — as I've documented in my experience with the breast prosthesis — I do detest artificial things. But the salon was located within the cancer hospital, and one day I found myself wandering in to see what was involved. A very nice woman explained to me that matching the silver, grey, and black in my hair would be a challenge, but she'd try. She went off to select appropriate wigs, while I stared at the variety on display. I was particularly taken by a long blonde thing with shoulder-length curls. It was full bodied and bawdy. I looked a bit like the Cowardly Lion in it. I really had the attendant befuddled when I asked if she could cut the top a bit, spike it, and dye it bright orange. I never did get a wig, but the experience was delightful.

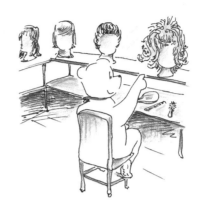

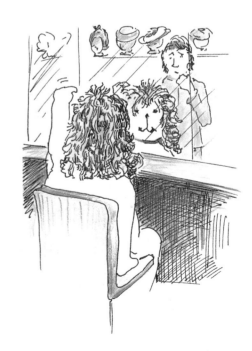

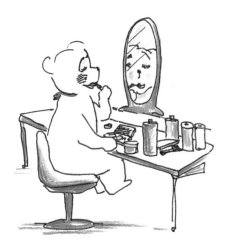

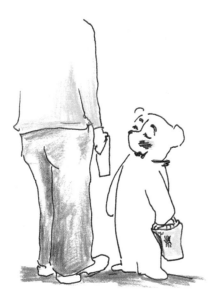

So too was the "Look Good, Feel Better" clinic. This is a program run by volunteers to help cancer patients, well … look good and feel better. Manufacturers donate a variety of wonderful products — makeup, lotions, nail treatments, soaps, and shampoos (we could always hope for hair again someday!) — to participants. A volunteer applied makeup to one half of my face, while I tried to copy her work on the other half. Her side looked ever so professional, while my side looked pretty pathetic. Nevertheless, I left the clinic with my package of donations and ran straight into my surgeon.

"How do I look?" I asked.

"Pretty good," he said.

"Then I must feel better!" I replied.

Chapter 18: In Which the Bear Has Even More Chemotherapy

Each round of chemo followed the same routine. Back to the hospital and to waiting in the blood clinic. (By the third treatment, I never wanted to see the hospital again.)

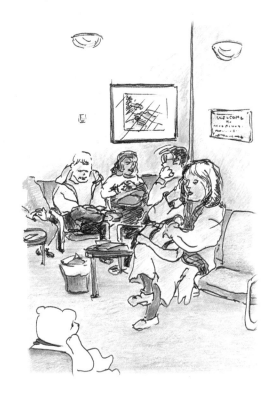

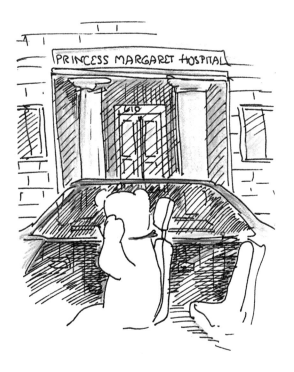

Back to the gynecological clinic. Back to waiting to see the specialist to find out whether my blood had recovered enough from the last treatment to go ahead with this one.

Back to the Day Care waiting room to ready myself for the treatment.

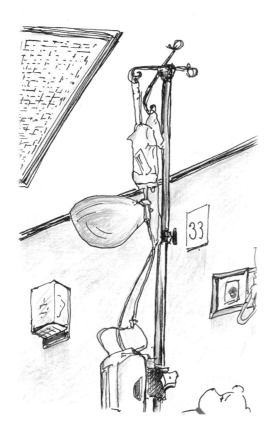

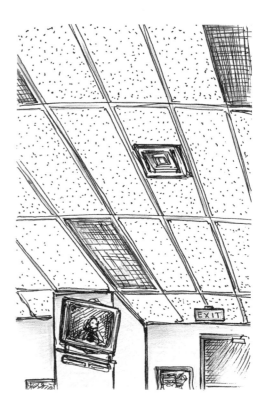

Back to the treatment room and its nauseating pink and green Naugahyde and bonging machines. Back to staring at ceilings.

And back to the hospital to get through
the worst of the treatment.

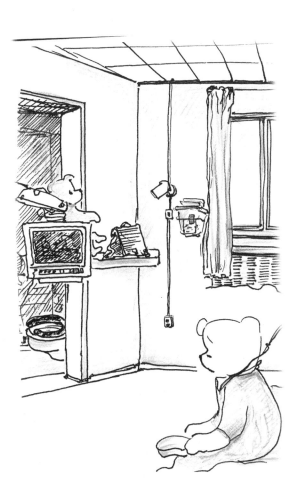

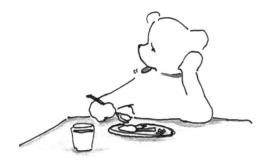

Then home, for more of the same: back to not being able get anything in, and not being able to get anything out, despite the many medications and solutions. How much rhubarb, flax, bran, prunes, and mineral oil would it take to counteract the side effects of the drugs?

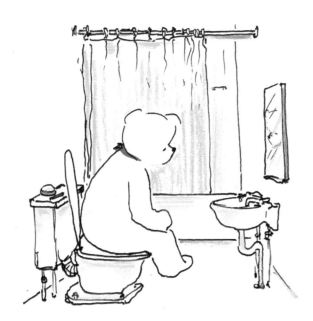

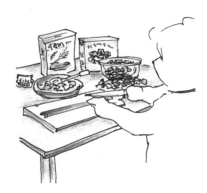

My friends appeared with casseroles and cupcakes and enticing dishes, hoping to inspire my insides to get back on track. When the refrigerator got overloaded, it was party time! Friends gathered to wine and dine on the tasty treats.

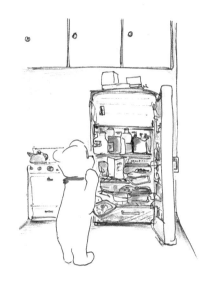

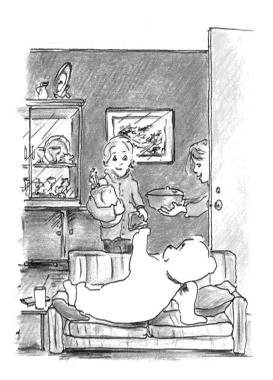

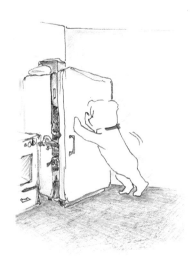

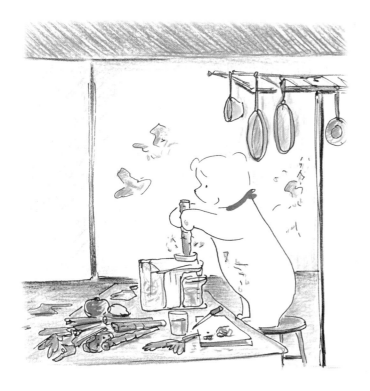

Then there were the joys of fresh juices. A friend loaned me her juicer so I could concoct my own carrot, apple, beet, and ginger juices, and combinations thereof. But the biggest drawback was cleaning the appliance. Good as the juices tasted, it took ten times longer to clean the machine than to drink them. After a few weeks, I returned the juicer.

My family doctor suggested I try
acupuncture. This experiment lasted
about four months longer than the juicer.

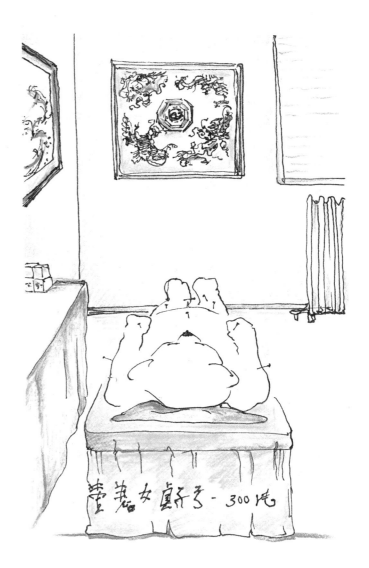

THE DAYS JOAN BREWED ESSIAC

BOIL
SIMMER
STAND
BOIL
SIMMER
STAND
REFRIGERATE
POUR
STAND
POUR AGAIN
STAND

One of the nurses suggested I try Essiac, a tea consisting of herbs like sheep sorrel, slippery elm, and burdock root, derived from an old Ojibwa recipe designed to boost the immune system. A dear friend took it upon herself to produce this concoction for me, a project that required extensive time: sterilizing containers and utensils, followed by hours of boiling, simmering, standing, straining, boiling again, and so forth, all to obtain a liquid that tasted like hay and was to be consumed in two-ounce quantities every twelve hours. We persevered with the Essiac for more than a year, long enough to give it a good try. As my tumour marker rose, however, indicating increased gremlin activity, my confidence in Essiac fell away.

The chemo was taking its toll on my energy, my hair, and my memory. I saw a study on television linking memory loss to toxicity levels of chemotherapy. I was sure that soon I wouldn't remember a thing. At least I had an excuse beyond senility for confusing words and forgetting things.

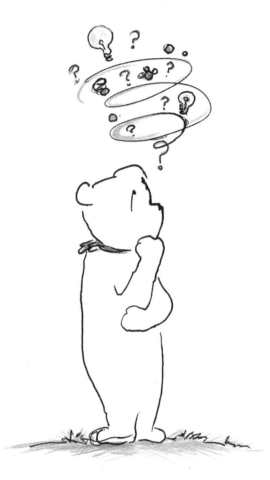

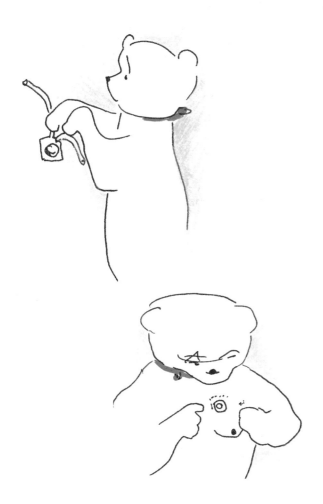

By the fourth chemo treatment, most of the veins in my left arm were unusable. Because of the mastectomy, my right arm couldn't be used either. It was time to implant a "portacath," a titanium device with a silicon centre and a long plastic tube that is inserted into a major vein to the heart. The whole device is positioned in the upper chest, implanted just beneath the skin so nurses can access the silicon port to extract blood or administer chemo drugs. I awoke from this operation to discover that the portacath projected about three-quarters of an inch out from my chest. Here I was, I joked, with my first "silicon implant" — and the surgeons had put it on the same side as my only breast. Now I had two little bumps on that side!

Every month now, I have to go to the hospital to have the portacath cleaned so it won't clog or be troublesome. And every month the nurses greet me with, "Are you here for a flush?" "Yes," I say, feeling like a toilet.

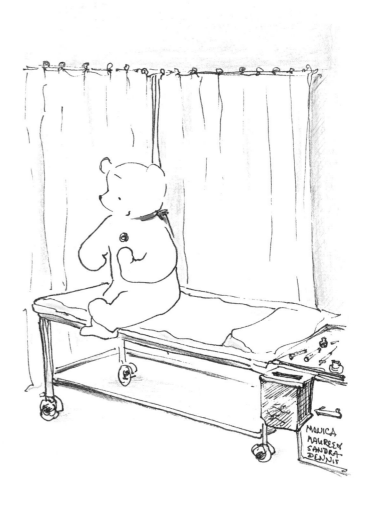

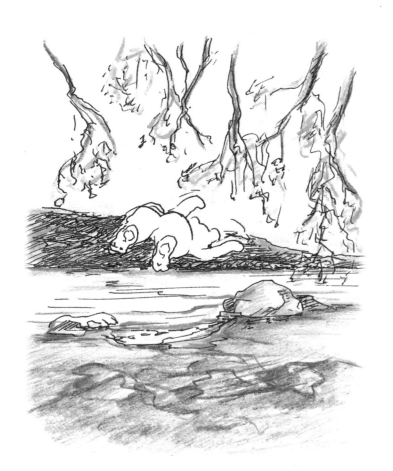

Chapter 19: In Which the Bear's CA 125 Count Rises

What a joy to finish the six months of chemo! I went back to the lake, looking forward to swimming, sailing, playing tennis, and eating and drinking and peeing and pooping, the simple basics of living.

I began drawing my bear, and contem-
plated turning the drawings and stories into
a publication that could serve as a fundraiser
for ovarian cancer and provide information
to other women experiencing the disease.
Life seemed filled with promise. I felt
stronger every day.

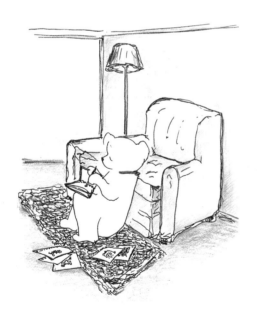

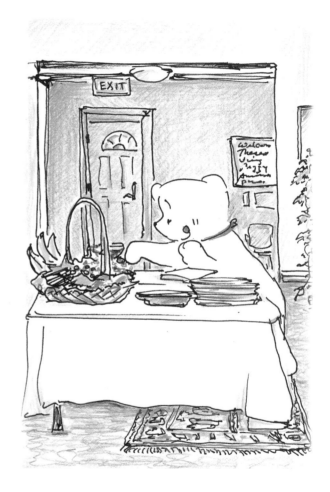

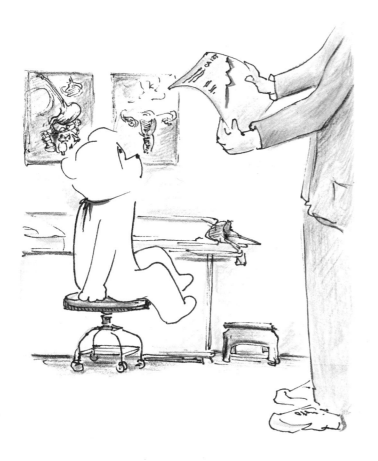

So how could my CA 125 count be on the rise? This count is a "tumour marker" that can be a fairly accurate indicator of tumour activity related to ovarian cancer — at least in some patients. It has been a fairly accurate indicator in my case. Before my most recent operation, the count had been in the thousands. The surgery and chemo had reduced it to nearly zero. But now, with each blood test, the counts began edging their way up.

Sometimes, the cancer gremlins seemed to stall, and occasionally the count dropped slightly. Whenever that happened, the nurses would call to tell me the good news and suggest that I keep doing whatever I was doing. They were so supportive.

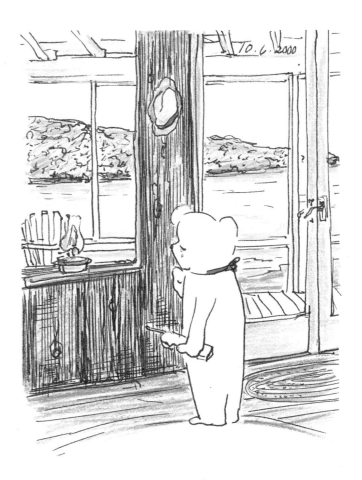

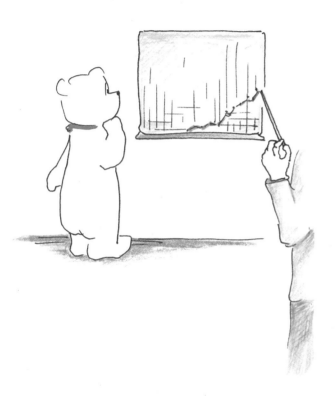

But, overall, the count kept rising. I looked at my chart and wished it could have been the stock market instead of my CA 125 levels. I thought about how stupid the cancer cells were. Didn't they realize that if I died, they died too?

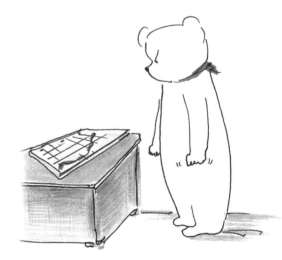

After several months, I was pronounced "symptomatic," which meant it was time to have more ultrasounds and CAT scans to review the situation. So much for all that juice and tea and acupuncture and good living!

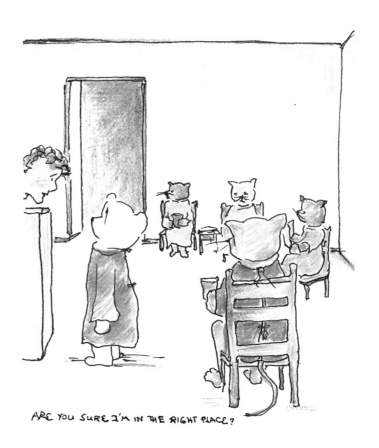

ARE YOU SURE I'M IN THE RIGHT PLACE?

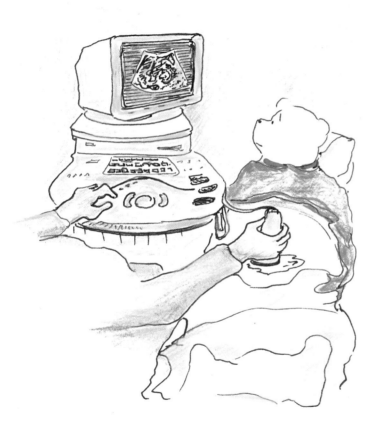

This time, the technician positioned the screen of the monitor so I could follow the ultrasound scan while she typed information into the keyboard. I saw what looked like one of the tumours. They were starting to develop in the lymph nodes surrounding the aorta.

"So, is that the largest tumour?" I asked.

"Yes, it is," she replied.

"Could you hit 'delete'?"

She looked and me and grinned. "Nobody has ever asked that before!"

"How about 'cut and send to trash'?"

"I wish I could," she told me. "I wish I could."

Chapter 20: In Which the Bear Trudges Back to Chemo

Once again it was time to consider how to fight the little gremlins on the rampage. My gynecological oncologist/surgeon advised a relatively conservative route: six more months of chemotherapy, this time using only the drug Carboplatin.

And so it was back to the clinics,

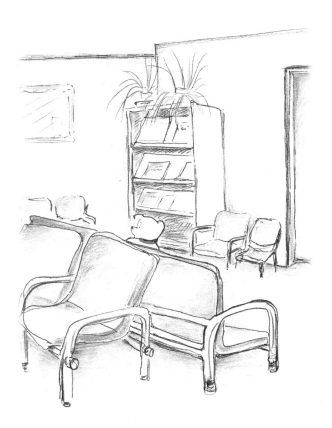

back to the Day Care,

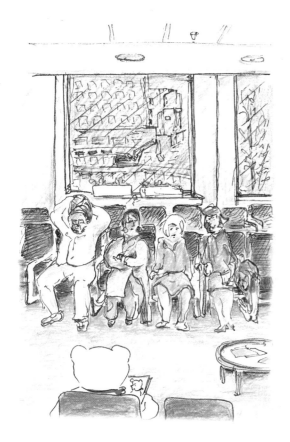

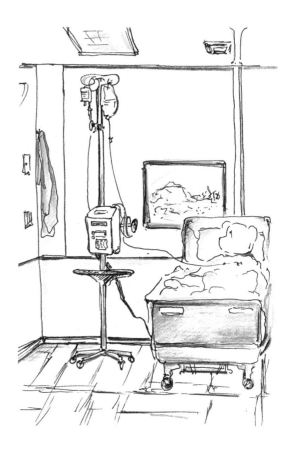

and back to the treatment centre.

Back to boring ceilings, bonging regulators,
and plastic bags of various toxins hanging
from IV poles. I couldn't imagine how the
staff coped when ten or twelve regulators
all went off at the same time, demanding
attention.

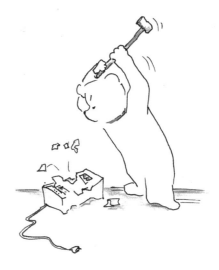

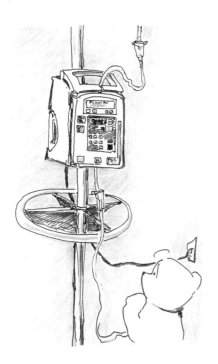

I wanted to kill those machines!
And I could have done a job on all
those hanging bags, too.

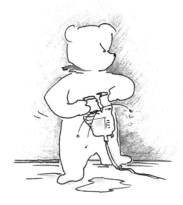

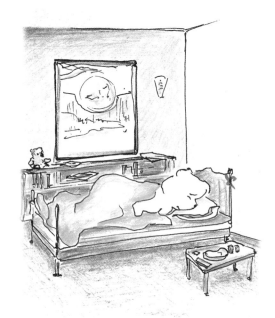

For six more months, I endured the side effects caused by the treatments. For a period of time I couldn't eat. And, once again, it was nearly impossible to get anything out. I spent so much time on the toilet I'm surprised it didn't leave a permanent impression on my behind.

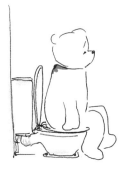

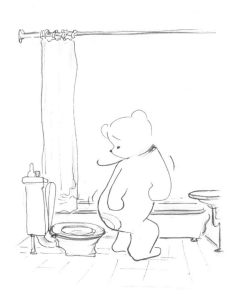

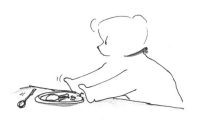

Each month, from December 2000 to
June 2001, chemo dashed my energy. As
often as possible, I returned to my "healing
place" to rebuild my spirits. Those six months
were followed by four wonderful months
drawing, sailing, swimming, and building
up strength in between hospital visits to check
my blood and flush the portacath.

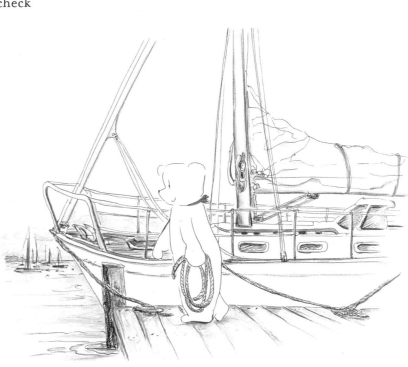

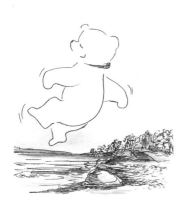

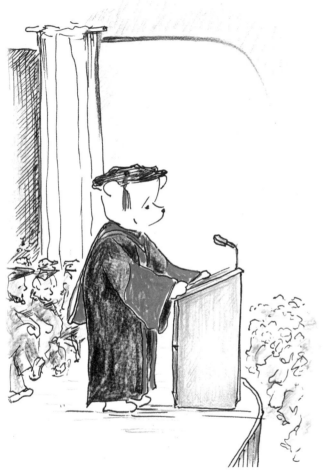

My college honoured me by selecting me as the commencement speaker. My presentation, titled "Life Is a River — Dam(n)," seemed to be well received.

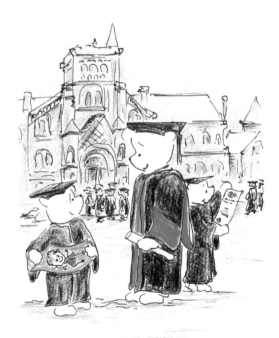

Unfortunately, come September, my CA 125 levels had risen significantly. Scans indicated a worsening in appearance of the retroperitoneal metastatic lymph nodes.

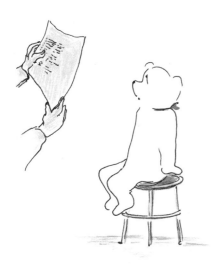

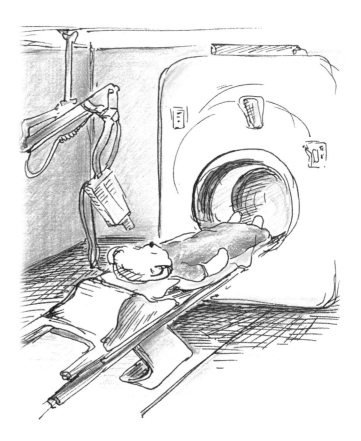

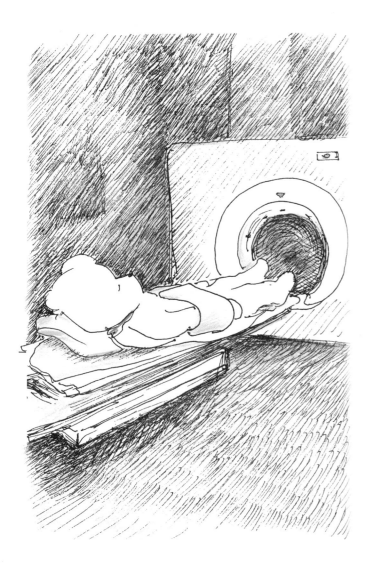

In October, I had a positron emission tomography (PET) scan, in which the more active cells "light up" on the monitor and offer insights as to the location of abnormal cell activity. The little gremlins seemed to have concentrated in an area in front of my L3 vertebra and to the right of the L2 vertebra.

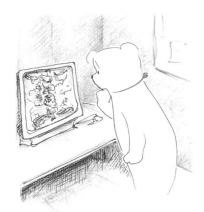

My special surgeon/oncologist and I agreed upon a somewhat radical approach: go for a couple more months of chemo in an attempt to shrink the tumours, making them less "sticky" and more readily operable, and follow with a laparotomy (to remove periaortic lymph nodes), more chemo, and perhaps radiation.

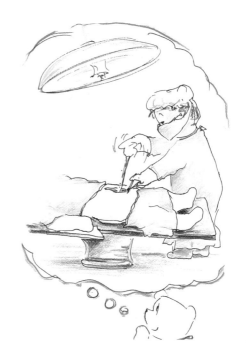

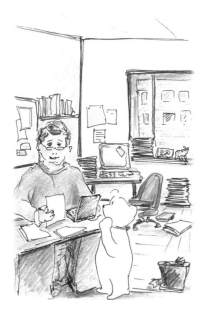

"This won't be curative," he said, "but if we're successful, it will get you more time!"

I was all for more time. I hadn't yet completed this book. I figured I'd probably get a few more bear chapters out of the experience.

So we were on course for more chemo, more surgery, and more time!

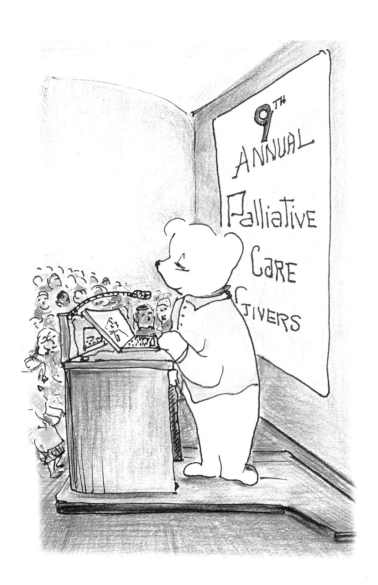

In April of 2002, the National Ovarian
Cancer Association asked me to be a part
of their first ever Ovarian Symposium, in
Toronto. I gave a lecture called "Bearing Up
with Cancer," and told my story, illustrated
with slides of the bear. I got a standing
ovation. I began lecturing at all of the
NOCA's symposia and to other organiza-
tions, travelling to St. John's, Winnipeg,
Vancouver, Halifax, Calgary, and the United
States to talk about the bear's experiences.
I also talked to doctors, nurses, and donors,
and to the ninth annual conference for
palliative care givers. I told them that they
were the most appropriate audience for me
at that particular time: I had just come from
spending the weekend in the hospital for my
last round of chemotherapy — if I threw up,
I said, I was sure they'd feel right at home.

My mother once said, "You know, Annie, if you live long enough, you live longer!" At the time, I remember thinking it was a pretty dumb statement. But I now see great wisdom in that remark. As geneticists, biologists, oncologists, and the various specialists in all medical fields share knowledge and research worldwide, they give us great hope. My Mom died of ovarian cancer in the early 1980s. Two decades later, I wish that the resources available to me had been hers.

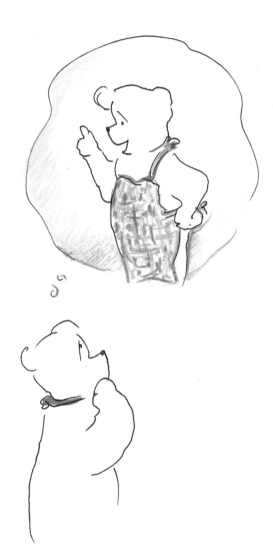

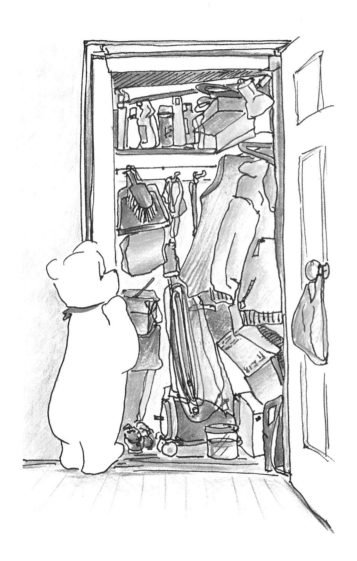

Chapter 21: In Which the Bear Has Yet Another Operation

I often have good intentions about not leaving things to the last minute, but I seldom succeed. Thus I found myself with a mountain of tasks the day before my surgery was scheduled. I wanted to meet with the future editor of the bear book, meet with my lawyer and a witness to finalize my will, answer some important correspondence, pay some bills, clean the closet, and make several phone calls. On top of all that, I was not to eat. At noon, I was to take an internal cleansing potion that, as it turned out, not only cleansed the bowel but also left me vomiting for several hours.

Fortunately the editor came in the morning, before potion time, and we had an uninterrupted discussion.

"Now, Annie," she said, "I have to ask a gloomy question."

"Yes?"

"Well, if something should happen to you, how do you wish the book to end?"

"Excellent question! How about 'rudely interrupted'!" I suggested.

Fortunately as well, my lawyer and her witness came in the late afternoon, by which time the ferociousness of the potion was more bearable. The will got signed, bills were paid, and correspondence was answered, as were the many phone calls. I never got around to cleaning the closet, though.

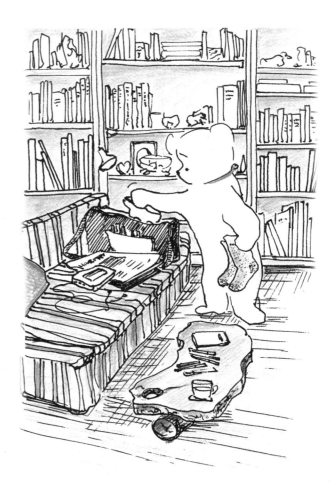

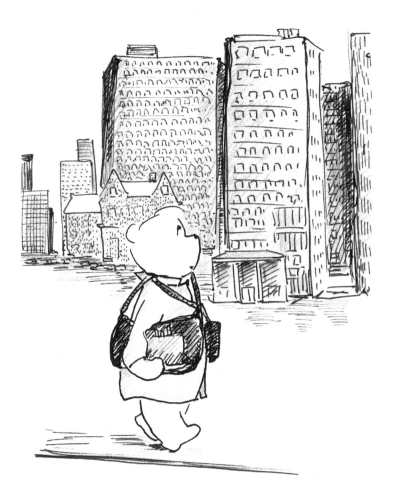

I arrived at the hospital at six the morning of the surgery and underwent the usual preparations: checking a blood sample for granulation, being injected with a shot of the blood thinner heparin, donning a hospital gown, taking the elevator to the surgical floor, lying on a stretcher in the holding room, being covered with a warm blanket, chatting with the anesthesiologist, and being wheeled into the OR. At my request, my surgeon had brought in a camcorder to videotape the operation. I wanted more information for my bear drawings.

And I wanted to document my latest surprise for my surgical team, once more taped to my abdomen and concealed under my hospital gown. I'd wanted to treat the team to dinner at a Bavarian restaurant — except that I had planned to pen in a name change on the gift certificate to make it read "Ovarian Restaurant." To my disbelief, however, all the Bavarian restaurants in the city had either become trendy bistros or had gone out of business. I chose what I thought to be the next best thing — a restaurant called Juice for Life. A gift certificate for that and a drawing of the bear on the operating table with IV bags filled with grape, carrot, kiwi, and various other kinds of juice completed the surprise.

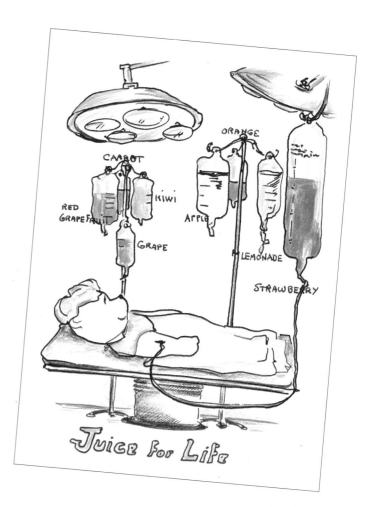

Chapter 22: In Which the Post-operative Bear Has Some Adventures

One of my earliest post-surgery recollections is my surgeon in the hospital room. He was all smiles as he reported that the operation had gone really well.

"There's even dialogue on the tape with me holding the large tumour and saying, 'Here it is, Annie, here's the big one!' I just wish the nurse had held the camcorder a bit higher."

Then he told me I'd been cut from stem to stern, sliced and diced, and I should do nothing but rest for a few days. Unfortunately, resting for a few days would prove harder than I expected.

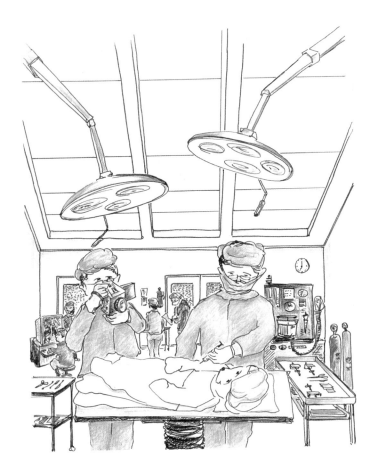

A naso-gastric tube carried bile and liquids from my stomach out through my right
nostril. An oxygen tube passed over my ears
and into both nostrils. The roof of my mouth
and the back of my throat were uncomfortably
irritated. The surgical dressing over the
stitches felt flat (no rings this time). A Foley
catheter was in place, and the IV tube for
saline, drugs, and morphine was still in my
right arm. The backs of my heels ached.
My vision was blurred due to the anesthetic
drugs. And I was unbelievably thirsty — I
wasn't even allowed ice chips. I headed into
a long, sleepless night.

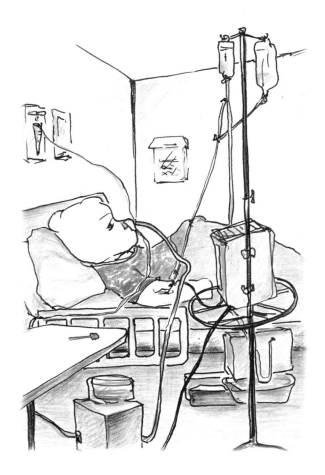

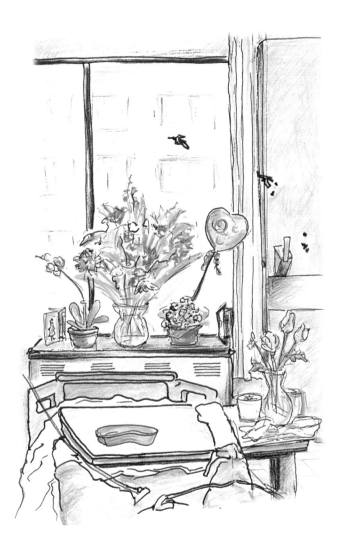

By the light of morning I was aware that my blurred vision was infused with floating black dots, some of which were so large that I thought they were pigeons flying by my window until they passed over the curtains and onto the wall. I was given moist swabs to bathe my mouth, and I was allowed tiny flakes of ice.

All in all, things went quite well until mid-morning, when a second-year nursing student from a nearby college was assigned to me. I knew I was in trouble when it took her four attempts to position the blood-pressure cuff on my arm and three readings to make sure of the results. Her insistence on bathing me — and on disconnecting the IV tube in order to remove my hospital gown — was most unfortunate. Nobody could reconnect the IV: not the student, her teacher, a nurse practitioner on the floor, or my own RN. Six hours later — six hours without saline, drugs, or morphine — a special IV nurse qualified to transfer the whole IV apparatus over to the portacath managed to restore the connection.

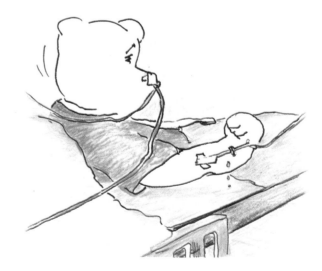

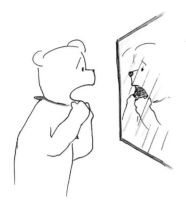

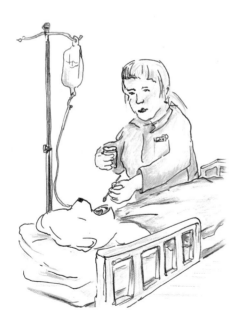

By Day 6, recovery was progressing slowly but steadily. I'd been up and walking since the day after my operation (mostly because the second-year nursing student had removed the catheter too early, forcing me to walk to the washroom) and I was registering ten – great guns – on the incentive spirometer. The naso-gastric tube had been removed on Day 4, and I looked a lot more attractive without all that green bile passing through the tube in my nose. I was allowed to try clear liquids, only to discover that the roof of my mouth had been badly cut by the insertion of the endotracheal tube and had ulcerated. A small glitch, but I now needed nursing assistance to apply the anesthetizing lidocaine hydrochloride to the sores and to take care not to drip the medication to my throat and cause paralysis.

That day, I noticed that the bag of saline solution had run dry. The head nurse and her colleague, acting on advice from the IV experts, attempted to start the portacath flowing again. They were to insert a syringe, draw it back until blood was extracted, then slowly push the blood and saline solution back through the line to reactivate the flow. The blood that appeared, however, looked odd, as if there were bubbles in it. When the gentle pushing started, I felt a sudden pain. Putting my hand to my neck, I discovered a golf-ball sized blowup in the jugular vein, the entry point for the tube from the portacath. Oh-oh. Everything stopped. The resident doctor was called, followed by a young doctor from vascular surgery, a portable X-ray machine to check for a break or blockage in the line, and two doctors from general surgery.

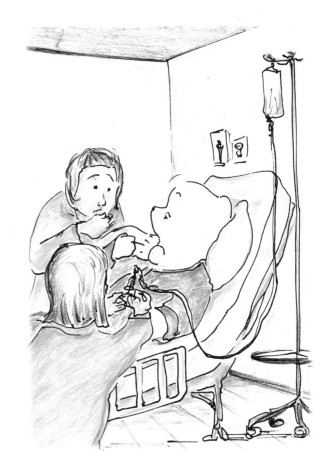

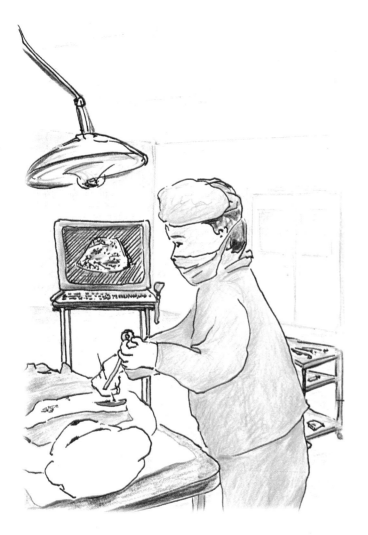

After much fuss, I was taken to interventional radiology, where the portacath was replaced. This time it was embedded more deeply and inserted on the right side, so my new silicon implant ended up balancing the other breast after all.

As long as I was in the hospital, it seemed appropriate to start another course of Carboplatin, followed with a few days of hydration and anti-nausea drugs. I'm not sure why, but I felt I handled this chemo regime better than I had any of the others. Perhaps the usual effects of the chemo seemed to pale in the light of all else I had endured.

On postoperative Day 11, my nurse allowed me to use the special scissors to remove the flat staples, thirty-six in all, from my incision. The IV specialist from the twelfth floor disconnected me from my IV pole. I was no longer on a "leash," and I was discharged — at least until the next round of chemotherapy.

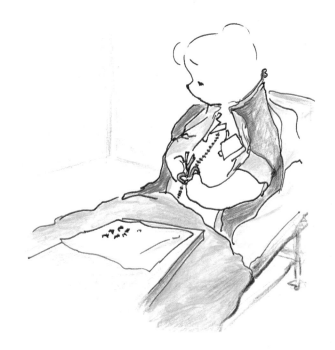

It was a beautiful, sunny day. Very few leaves showed on the trees, but the smell of spring filled the air.

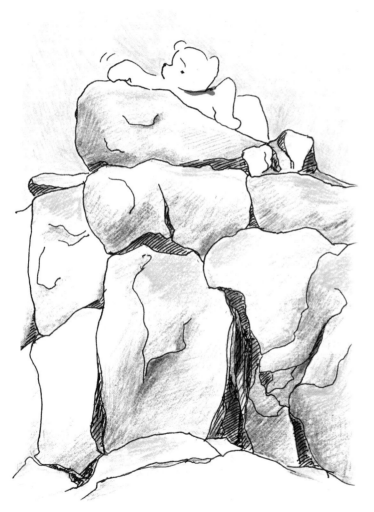

Epilogue: In Which the Bear Is Not Quite Rudely Interrupted

My journey with cancer isn't over yet — as I write this, my doctors are considering radiation, and there are always more scans and blood tests to keep me occupied.

But we all know how the story will end.

I never have been good at facing death. I'm very sentimental. I tear up at parades and the playing of the national anthem. I cried when the Canadian men's and women's hockey teams won the Olympic gold in 2002. Friends shield me from movies they think would upset me. All my life, my Mom urged me to "get ahold of myself," to straighten up, grow up, and better learn to handle death, sadness, and injustices, or joys and exhilaration — whatever touched my soul.

Medicine consoles me. I haven't yet had a doctor give up on me. I have confidence in the medical profession and its abilities to help me confront this disease again and again — and again. And I keep reminding myself that, after all, it is only a disease. It can be confronted. I am a doctor of philosophy, but I sometimes find myself frustrated that I am not also a medical doctor. I wonder whether I would be better able to handle death and dying if I had become one. I don't think so.

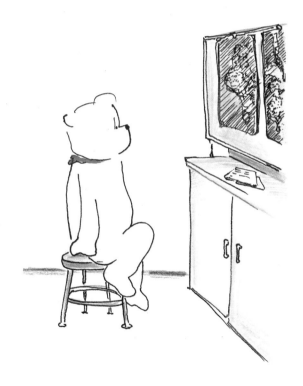

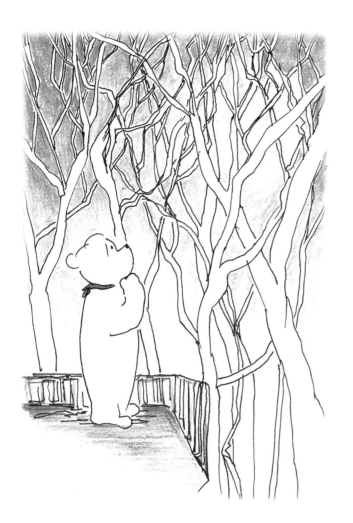

Nature consoles me. Being alone at my barn on its lake — my "healing place" — is sometimes my best medicine. I sit out on a point and stare at the ever-changing waters that have been a part of my life since childhood. With every new phase in my efforts against those gremlins, I try to feel strong, but I have my moments. I stare at the sky and water, study the trees and tangle of limbs, and I wonder when the leaves will start to bud and how and where I'll be when that happens. No one sees the tears. No one tries to comfort me and tell me to be brave when I wonder whether being brave makes any difference.

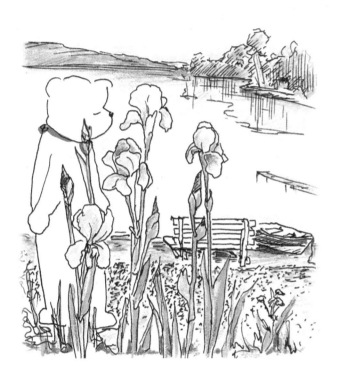

Medical answers to our private questions about living and dying have to do with statistics. Along with so many others involved with cancer, I have had to listen to my share of bad news. But from the very first notices, I remember telling the physicians, "Someone has to be on the positive side of all those negative numbers. Someone has to be on the good side and it might as well be me!"

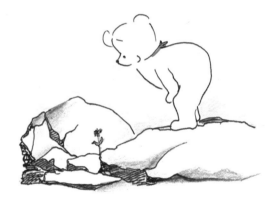

I have been saying that since 1984, when
I first began to confront the cancer gremlins.
Nearly two decades later, I know I can't
control the future, but I think I've defied
the odds. More than anything, I know that
I have truly lived each minute
of the last nineteen years.
I have truly lived with
cancer — and that sure
beats dying.

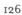